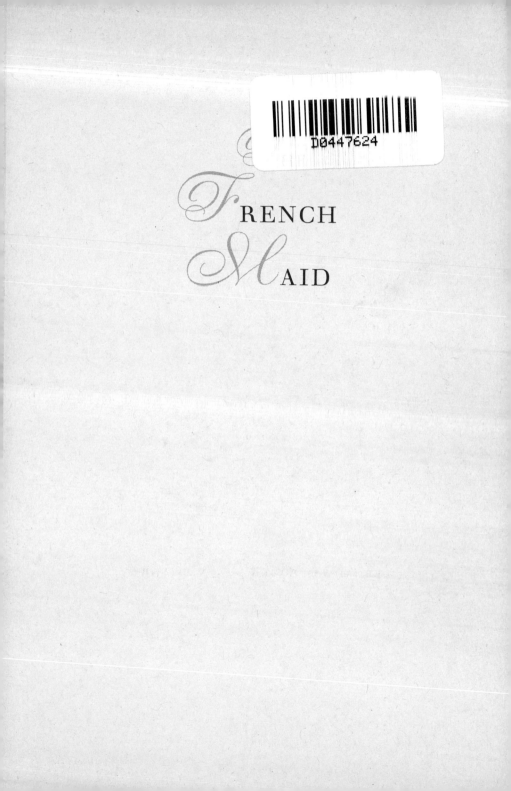

FRENCH MAID

BROADWAY BOOKS ⁓ NEW YORK

THE FRENCH MAID

And 21 More Naughty Sex Fantasies to Surprise and Arouse Your Man

DON & DEBRA MACLEOD

BROADWAY

THE FRENCH MAID. Copyright © 2005 by Don and Debra Macleod.
All rights reserved. No part of this book may be reproduced or transmitted
in any form or by any means, electronic or mechanical, including photocopying,
recording, or by any information storage and retrieval system, without
written permission from the publisher. For information, address
Broadway Books, a division of Random House, Inc.

PRINTED IN THE UNITED STATES OF AMERICA

BROADWAY BOOKS and its logo, a letter B bisected on the diagonal,
are trademarks of Random House, Inc.

Visit our website at www.broadwaybooks.com

First edition published 2005

Book design by Caroline Cunningham

Library of Congress Cataloging-in-Publication Data
Macleod, Don, 1971–
The French maid : And 21 more naughty sex fantasies
to surprise and arouse your man /
Don Macleod, Debra Macleod.— 1st ed.
p.   cm.
1. Sex instruction for women. 2. Sexual fantasies. 3. Sexual excitement.
I. Macleod, Debra, 1969–   II. Title.
HQ46.M185 2005
613.9'6—dc22   2004045936

ISBN 0-7679-1786-3

1 3 5 7 9 10 8 6 4 2

This book is dedicated to each other, with much love.

Who says research can't be fun?

CONTENTS

ACKNOWLEDGMENTS

MANY THANKS to Jimmy at the Vines Agency, and to Kristine Puopolo and Elizabeth Haymaker at Broadway Books for their invaluable editorial direction.

The French Maid

INTRODUCTION

$\mathcal{L}$AST NIGHT, your partner climbed into the same bed he did the night before, pulled the same sheets over his body, turned off the same bedside lamp, and kissed the same woman good-night. It's his world, his reality, and he's used to it.

But tonight, he's in for a surprise. Tonight, he's leaving the real world behind, and stepping into the exhilarating world of sexual fantasy. Everything is different here. The look and feel of the room, the scent of the woman, and the softly enticing words being whispered into his ear. Especially different are the powerful, erotic images that flash across his mind's eye and arouse his body.

He is listening to a story—an erotic fantasy. But it's more than that. He is *immersed* in the fantasy. Perhaps the sheets are new, or the bedroom is lit by a candle. Perhaps unusual music is playing. The woman lying next to him is also unfamiliar. She moves differently, sounds different, and touches him in a different way. He can easily believe he is somewhere else, *with* someone else. It is sexually intoxicating.

In *The French Maid*, we take sexual fantasy to new heights using the power of erotic storytelling. Our goal is to bring the excitement of variety, the thrill of the unfamiliar, and the lure of the forbidden into a committed relationship. *The French Maid* lets you be every woman to your man!

We've designed the fantasies in this book to be initiated and told by a woman to her partner. (If male readers rise up and demand a book of fantasies to "surprise and arouse" their women, we'll be happy to oblige.) For your convenience, each fantasy is presented fully scripted, complete with dialogue and comprehensive directions for steamy sexplay. While some fantasies may benefit from a simple prop, all can be enjoyed without. You may like the idea of dressing the part, and we encourage you to do so, but it is certainly not necessary. We've written the book so that you can simply whisper the fantasy in your partner's ear as you get physical. His imagination—and yours—will do the rest.

However, we do suggest simple changes that will help transport your partner to the fantasy world, and make him experience his real world and his real woman in a new way. Change the color of a lightbulb in a room. Serve movie food for dinner on paper plates. And to make a new you? Apply a temporary tattoo to your breast or your bottom. Change the way you move or sound during sex. If you're usually loud, surprise him with silence. If you're usually quiet, this time moan at his every touch. Each fantasy in *The French Maid* comes with its own story-specific suggestions. They're quick and easy changes you can plan today, to have exciting results tonight.

Each love scene begins with a brief outline of its plot and suggestions for how you might want to ease into it or set it up. For simplicity, all dialogue—everything you will say to your partner—is italicized. As the fantasy proceeds, dialogue is interspersed with action; that is, physical directions, suggestions, sexual techniques, and other sexy tidbits you may wish to include while you speak.

Of course, you will not need to memorize each and every word of dialogue—good storytellers never do. Remember that the goal is to have sex, not to study! But do be sure to bring a good working knowledge of the fantasy's contents with you when you climb into bed. Reading the fantasy in advance a couple of times should do it. You will absorb enough of the details, directions, and dialogue to present a great fantasy and have lots of fun. So be playful, and use artistic license whenever you or your partner wants to.

Reading these fantasies will give you a definite sense of where to begin, what to do, and what to say, but use your own discretion and don't feel you must blindly adhere to the script. We all have physical and emotional limits that only we can be the judge of. If you're not sure whether you have the comfort level to act out a scene, say a word, or accept a particular aspect of a fantasy, simply omit it or substitute it with something else.

At the same time, you might want to consider that people's sexual fantasies are rarely politically or morally correct. Some of the fantasies in *The French Maid* involve a degree of reluctance or unawareness on the part of one partner or the other, and two involve sex with very young women. Nearly every fantasy involves sex between near-strangers. Whether or not you approve of these things in real life, in the world of fantasy and in the private moments between you and your loving partner, enjoying what might be wrong is nothing to be ashamed of. It is a fact of human sexuality that the forbidden can be extremely arousing, and it is the reason erotic fantasies are so popular. They provide the perfect outlet to explore the frontiers of your sexual imagination, consensually and harmlessly.

The fantasies in this book are explicit and often edgy. You and your partner may not get through an entire fantasy at once, so you can return repeatedly, going a little further each time. Many provide options, so again you can return to the same fantasy, but play it out differently. You may find that you use the stories simply as foreplay, or that you stop in the middle of a fantasy and let nature take its course. If you do get off track but want to keep the spirit of the fantasy alive during your lovemaking, there are short "sexy snippets" included at the end of each fantasy—whisper these into your partner's ear, and you won't miss a beat. Or you can memorize a few of your own favorite lines from the fantasy.

The fantasies here are ones that we thought would arouse most men by capitalizing on that which is forbidden. But even if they begin with male pleasure in mind, female pleasure is never secondary or incidental. Since you are the storyteller, you can direct much of the fantasy to satisfy your own sexual desires, as well as what you know of his.

The fantasy world is best enjoyed when partners share a confident and open-minded acceptance of each other's sexuality, and a willingness to help each other explore it with en-

thusiasm. There is no doubt in our minds that sexual enthusiasm can cancel out any real or imagined damage that
Time's gravitational pull, your pregnancies, or simply the ill
will of the gods has done to your body. As women, we often
deprive ourselves unnecessarily, whether it is by keeping the
lights off, shunning sexy nighties, or even skipping positions
we think aren't flattering. Once you've tried a fantasy or two,
you'll see how quickly all those little flaws fade to black when
the sexual imagination catches fire.

Finally, remember that variety is the spice of life—and of
sex. Season these fantasies to your taste, and dig in.

1

MORE THAN MASSAGE

ANY MEN have fantasized about a massage getting a little out of control and becoming sexual.
Who can blame them? The feeling of skin on skin and the
deep, repetitive strokes are both soothing and stimulating at
the same time. The fact that the masseuse is so close, yet so
off-limits, is very arousing. Therefore, this is a situation that
can easily cause a man's mind to wander and his thoughts to
quickly turn sexual. In this fantasy, your partner is the unsuspecting but serendipitous client of a very ambitious—and
amorous—massage artist.

If you have never played with sexual fantasies before, this
is the perfect "first" fantasy to lead him through. It starts
with an innocent back rub, and effortlessly progresses into a
very erotic fantasy situation. Because it unfolds so naturally,
you don't have to stress over how to make the transition from
reality into fantasy. He'll never suspect that you had this ex-

perience planned. Also, this fantasy is relatively tame compared to some of the others in this book; there is no "dirty talk" and the storyline is straightforward. It will ease you into using fantasies in your sex life.

After your partner accepts your offer of a back rub, ask him to lie on his belly and then straddle his back. Make sure you're not wearing panties underneath your nightie. You want him to feel the nakedness between your legs when you climb on top of his back. This may surprise and arouse him in itself. Use a nicely scented lotion or oil to rub his back, but scented just enough that he will notice. A musk scent is great to set the mood for massages, and a favorite of many men.

Lean over and light a candle. Remember that a candle has the power to transform any dark room into a massage parlor. As an alternative, replace the white lightbulb in your bedside lamp with a red one. It may also be a nice touch to have preset the radio by your bed to a classical station, or to another favorite that offers relaxing music. If you are really committed, you can put new satin sheets on your bed to further contrive the ambiance of a massage parlor. Do what you need to transport your partner to the fantasy world, by making your bedroom look and feel a little different than it usually does. This will help immerse both of you into your "roles."

Begin the massage by rubbing his shoulders, all the way down his arms and to his hands. He might also enjoy having his scalp massaged or stimulated with a stiff-bristled brush. Give him some time to relax and settle into the soothingly repetitive motions of your strokes. Up until now you've probably just been talking about work or the kids, if you have any, but now you can begin to ease into a more sexual conversation that will give you an opportunity to slip into fantasy mode.

You can say something like:

Did you ever wonder what happens behind closed doors in some of those seedy little massage parlors? You know the ones. They're just off the street downtown, usually down a dirty flight of stairs. I can imagine what they look like inside... rows of private cubicles with heavy curtains drawn around them.

You want to get your partner thinking about this and letting his mind wander in more erotic directions. You want him to clearly visualize the type of place you're describing. No doubt the conversation will take on a life of its own surrounding the goings-on inside some massage parlors, but remember to keep rubbing and stroking his back all the while.

Lift yourself off his back, turn yourself around, and lower yourself down again so that you're facing his foot. Keep massaging his buttocks and legs as far down as you can reach while the two of you continue to talk about the less reputable massage parlors in town. Lean over and press yourself into his skin. Let him feel you getting wet against his back.

Turn yourself around again, and begin to grind yourself into his lower back and upper buttocks with more force and urgency.

Mmmm, that feels good... have you ever imagined what it would be like to get a massage in a place like that? I wonder if the girls ever want to climb on top of their customers, like this? I'll bet a lot of them do.

Pull your nightie off over your head. Lean forward so that he can feel your breasts against his back. Communicate your pleasure by moaning softly, since the sound of sexual excitement is arousing in itself. It is also important to remember to keep moving. Keep brushing your skin against his, sometimes so softly that only your nipples touch his back, and sometimes more strongly. Remember that you're an agile, lustful masseuse, so get into the role. Your partner will love feeling the movement of your body on top of his, and you will enjoy touching him this way.

Try to cover the whole surface of his back, even reaching behind yourself to stroke his buttocks. The more surface area of his skin that you can stimulate, the better. Vary your motions, too. When you are leaning forward, lightly kiss and lick his back. Drag your fingertips down it with a light, feathery touch, all the while rocking and letting him feel your wetness on his back.

Now start to be more specific about where he is and what is happening to him. Help him visualize himself as an active participant in this fantasy by providing clear descriptions, and by leading him step by step through the plot.

Say something like:

Imagine you're in one of those places, in the little private cubicle, lying on a thin massage bed. The curtains are drawn around you. Your body is being massaged and rubbed with long, firm strokes. Your eyes are closed and you're lost in your own relaxed thoughts. You don't even notice that her strokes are becoming more sexual.

Imagine that all of a sudden the masseuse climbs on top of you like this. You can feel she's already wet, and the moment she straddles your back she gets even wetter. You know she's enjoying it. And so are you. You don't know if you should say anything to her, but you have to be quiet, since there's only a curtain

separating you from the other customers and you don't want to
get caught…unless they're doing the same thing.

Lift yourself off your partner's back, and have him flip
over so he's lying on his back. Position yourself so that you
are sitting backward, facing his feet, with his genitals ahead
of you. Let him look at your bare back and behind first, since
he will be expecting to see your face. Again, lean over and rub
as far down his legs as you can, allowing him a close-up view
of your bare bum. Your belly will press against his genitals,
but don't massage them. Enjoy the idea of what you are doing, and the sensation of feeling your partner's body in what
may be a new way for you.

It will be a surprisingly erotic treat for your man if you
have applied a temporary tattoo to your lower back. This will
help engage his imagination and play to his sense of being in
another place with another body.

When you're ready, lift yourself off your partner and turn
around to face him. Lower yourself so that you are sitting
with his genitals behind you, just behind your bum. Remember that you have not yet touched his genitals with your
hands. His arms should be at his sides.

Sit straight up so that he can look at you, naked, for the
first time, straddling him. He should be able to look up and
luxuriate in the sight of your womanly form, so push your
shoulders back to make your breasts stand out. Continue to
move in a rocking motion, gyrating your wetness onto his
skin, and moaning to express your pleasure.

Reacquaint him with where he is and with what is happening to him.

Are you picturing yourself there? In a dirty little massage parlor? You just went in for a massage, maybe hoping in the back of your mind that the rumors about those places are true. At first the girl just rubbed you down, but then she couldn't help herself. She pulled off her robe and climbed on top of you, rubbing herself against you.

You know that nobody will find out. You can just enjoy how wrong and how dirty it is to be doing this. This woman will never tell. The cubicle is so dimly lit that you can hardly make out her face. You can't remember what she looked like when you first came in, but now she feels so exquisite that you don't care.

Caress his stomach and chest with your fingertips and gradually begin to massage the front of his body. Don't forget his arms and hands. Lift each hand into yours and massage it deeply. Take one of his fingers and put in it your mouth, sucking it. Make the most of this sensation by flicking your tongue around his finger and bobbing it in and out of your mouth.

I'll bet you taste wonderful.

Put his hand down and reach behind you. Caress his testicles and squeeze them softly. Move your hand lightly up and down the back of the shaft of his penis; but don't do this for too long since you just want to give him a taste of what is to come.

Lean forward and cover your partner's stomach and chest with soft kisses, moving your hands lightly over his skin at the same time. Let him feel your nipples and breasts press into him as you lean far forward to kiss his neck. Kiss all around his neck and ears, moving ever closer to his lips. Finally, kiss him deeply on his lips. Kiss him hard and desperately, using your tongue and sucking on his bottom lip. Stop suddenly.

Can I taste you down there?

Turn yourself around quickly, and in one motion take as much of his penis in your mouth as you can. Take it out just as quickly.

This girl wants to make you come.

Take his penis in your mouth again while tightly squeezing the sides of his body with your legs. Your partner should be able to enjoy the sight of your bum bent over him, while at the same time feeling your mouth move up and down his shaft and your legs squeeze his sides with sexual urgency. Make sounds of pleasure while you are performing oral sex so he knows you like it. Combining sights, sounds, and sensations will give you both the best sexual experience possible.

You will have to gauge how long you can perform oral sex on your man. If you want him to come while you are using your mouth, let him know it is okay for him to do so. Take your cues from him. If you want him to come inside you, or if you think he would prefer to, do not let him get too worked up during oral sex. Sit up, turn yourself around, and lower yourself onto his penis. As with most fantasies, you can satisfy your own sexual cravings by working them into the storyline.

This girl has to have you inside her, she can't stop herself... she doesn't care if she gets caught, she just wants to feel you fill her up. And it feels so good to you that you can't stop either. You can't think of anything but how good it feels to be inside this girl you don't know, and how she's moving up and down on your shaft while you just lie there. You can't believe this is really happening to you, and you can feel a strong orgasm building.

Have your man remain still while you move yourself up

and down his penis. Vary your speed; go slow and then fast and hard. Reach behind yourself and squeeze his testicles. Make sure he can tell by your moans and motions when you want to come and that you want him to come. By this point, it shouldn't take either one of you very long, and it should happen naturally.

You lie still as the orgasm takes over your body, and hers. The girl keeps moving up and down on you until your senses return. Finally, she climbs off the table. She cleans you with a warm, wet towel, then tells you that your time is up. You ask her how much you owe for the "extra," but she grins, and tells you it was her pleasure.

AFTERWARD, lie beside your partner and tell him how good he made you feel. Let him know how much fun you had with this fantasy, and that you hope he had fun too. Teasingly foreshadow that it won't be the last one. Bring him a hot facecloth and wipe his face, body, and genitals off. It will feel great when it cools on his skin. Bring him a glass of water. Without a doubt, your efforts will spring into his mind many times the next day, and he will begin to anticipate what you have in store for him the next time. And be sure to remember that the smile on your man's face is from thinking about you, not the shameless masseuse.

SEXY SNIPPETS

1. *All of a sudden, the girl climbs on top of you, straddling your back... you can feel she's a little wet.*

2. *The curtains are drawn in the little cubicle and the girl is lowering herself onto your shaft.*

3. *It feels so good and so wrong... you have to keep quiet or you'll get caught.*

4. *Nobody will ever find out, this girl will never tell.*

5. *The massage table is rocking as she bounces up and down on you in this dark little cubicle.*

2

EARLY-BIRD SWIMMING

THIS FANTASY is a great one for a lazy weekend morning. Many men feel especially frisky in the morning, so indulge your partner on occasion and flirt with him as the sun comes up. If he wakes up with an erection, playfully grab it and tell him you hope he was dreaming about you. Stroke his penis and his ego; the two are connected, in attitude if not anatomically. You'll set the tone for a great morning, and you'll provide a good reason for many shared secret smiles throughout the day.

Sex in the unforgiving light of day might be intimidating for you, but many men and women love it. To appease your reservations, make a quick visit to the bathroom to freshen up before your partner awakens. Wipe the sleep out of your eyes and brush your teeth. Climb back into bed before he wakes up, wearing only bikini bottoms or bikini-style panties.

If you really want to please him, surprise him by either removing or trimming your pubic hair. Many men and women appreciate the look and feel of smooth, hairless pubic area. Many men are also turned on by a variety of grooming styles in this area; shave or wax your pubic hair into a small rectangle, triangle, or stripe for a sexy change.

If you would rather, you can lead your partner through part or all of this fantasy under the shade of the sheets. While you're stroking him and telling him what a hot-blooded thoroughbred he really is, engage in a little conversational fiction.

Say something like:

Did you know that So-and-so goes to the pool for early-bird swimming a few times a week? He's probably there right now, swimming laps and swallowing chlorine. I'm not that ambitious.

Then whisper:

To tell you the truth, I think he has ulterior motives for going there. I think he's got a thing going with somebody there... who knows, maybe a bored lifeguard or a lonely housewife.

Now that you have so expertly directed your partner's mind, you can set the scene for him.

Imagine you go to early-bird swimming a few times a week. There's hardly anyone there at that hour, just you, a lifeguard that pops in and out of the pool area, and one or two other regulars.

Incorporate enough physical, sensory, and story details to bring the scene to life in your partner's sleepy mind.

Picture yourself just having arrived at the pool, and just coming out of the change room into the pool area. The tile floor is cold and wet, and the smell of chlorine fills your nostrils. The lifeguard chair is empty, as it usually is. There aren't enough people to worry about this early in the morning, so the life-guard takes a number of long coffee breaks. You don't care. The sound of your bare feet against the thin film of water on the tile floor echoes.

There's just you and one other person there. You recognize the woman at the other end of the pool... she's there most mornings that you're there. She's petite, with long dark hair. She's always wearing a black bikini, with white stars on the bra part. You've noticed she's fairly shapely, and she always smiles at you when she walks by. You've been brave enough to say "Hi" a few times, and she's always responded in a friendly way.

You climb down the ladder into the warm, turquoise water and begin to swim toward deeper water. You're lost in your own thoughts and, without realizing it, you've swam past the woman. She's going in the other direction, and you turn to follow her. For some reason, you feel a little rude that you haven't acknowledged her and you'd at least like to offer her a quick smile.

Begin to caress your partner's body. Wake him pleasantly with a light back-scratch, and run your fingers through his hair as you tell him your story.

You swim along leisurely behind her, and when you stop to get your bearings you're surprised to find that she's right in front of you. The water is just shallow enough that both of you can touch bottom, and you stand there dumbly for a moment, looking at each other. You offer a startled smile and she smiles back, more composed. You're stuck in an awkward situation and you're wondering how to get out of it... should you just swim away, should you say something, or wait for her to say something first?

You're considering your options when you notice something

floating just underneath the surface of the water in front of the woman. It's the top part of her bikini—it's come undone and she doesn't seem to know. You're mortified. Again you run through your options... should you just swim away and pretend you didn't notice, or should you discreetly point it out to her and hope she doesn't think you're a perv?

You try not to look directly at her breasts, but your eyes are automatically drawn there. You feel helpless as you stare shamelessly at her breasts, barely hidden just under the surface of the water. They're buoyed up by the water, and when she moves her arms a certain way, they lift above the surface so you can clearly see them. They're full and smooth, with small but erect dark nipples.

Tease your partner with a surprise early-morning glimpse of your naked breasts. He won't be expecting to see you barebreasted in the morning light, so this should rev him up even more.

The woman follows your gaze and realizes that her top is off and her breasts are exposed for a stranger to see. She doesn't react. In fact, she just looks up at you with a more intense smile. It's almost inviting. You feel yourself respond to her indiscretion and her flirting, and you hope she doesn't notice your erection under the water. Just as you're thinking this, she glides closer to you. You're shocked to feel her hand on your cock. She touches your hard-on and her smile grows even wider.

The woman moves her hands to her chest and cups a breast in each hand. She kneads them, and then pulls on them so the nipples are sticking out. She floats still closer to you and rubs her nipples against your body. She takes a fast look around the pool area, and after confirming that you are alone, she pushes her body up so that she is floating on her back.

You can see her breasts sticking out of the water, her nipples pointing to the ceiling. Your cock is getting harder by the second. The woman is floating on her back and you're admiring her beautiful curves and flawless skin. It's so strange to see a woman's naked body in this place, with the sounds echoing all around you, and the stark artificial lighting. She spreads her legs so you can see the crotch of her bikini bottom. You feel your cock pound as you reach between her legs and move the fabric to the side, giving you an unobstructed view of her. You find you're forgetting to breathe.

If you have trimmed your pubic hair, say something like:

You see folds of pink skin, and a small tuft of dark pubic hair that was hidden by her tiny bikini.

If you have removed your pubic hair completely, describe that by saying something like:

You see folds of pink skin, but no pubic hair. She looks smooth, soft, and perfect.

Continue to lead your partner through the fantasy while you stroke and caress his body. Direct his hand toward your panties and let him rub the fabric.

Feeling even braver, you look closely at her pussy as it floats toward you. You can see her slit and you feel an urge to finger it. You really want to know what she feels like.

As if in response, she opens her legs wider, presenting herself to you. You extend an anxious hand and tease her clit with a finger. You hear a moan echo throughout the pool area, and you're suddenly reminded of where you are.

Allow your partner to move your panties aside to make your vagina available to his touch. Direct his fingers toward your clitoris, and let him play with it. If you have removed your pubic hair, he will love the soft surprise. This can all be done under the covers if the brightness intimidates you, but do try to treat your partner to a view of your body in the morning light, if you can.

Refresh his visualization:

Imagine yourself in a pool with this stranger, a woman who has exposed her naked body to you. There's nobody else around, although they could return at any moment and you could get caught. The woman is floating on her back close to you, her breasts and erect nipples protruding out of the water.

Her legs are spread wide in front of you, and you're holding her bikini aside to look at her glistening pussy. You look down at your cock, and beneath the distortion of the water you can see it fully erect and hard. It's throbbing and aching.

Continue to lead your partner through the developing story.

The woman stands upright again. She looks at you devilishly, and you can tell she's thinking about fucking you, too. She gazes between your legs and then takes your hand. She pulls you toward her and wraps her legs around your body. She presses her pussy against you and the force of the contact jars your senses. Your cock aches from the attention, and you grind yourself against her.

Now do the same to your partner by pressing your groin against his penis.

You're concentrating on pushing yourself against her body, so you don't immediately notice that the lifeguard has returned. He's at the other end of the pool, putting some water toys into a big basket. It's moms-and-tots swimming next. The woman quickly refastens her bikini top and begins to swim away from you. You don't want her to go. You want more of that feeling of pressing up against this new, unfamiliar body, especially with the risky surroundings adding to your arousal.

You decide to pursue her and you swim after her. She glances behind, sees you following, and smiles broadly. When she reaches the ladder, she climbs out of the pool and heads for the family changing room instead of the ladies' changing room. You know why... it's because you won't be interrupted. There won't be anyone in there for at least a half hour, so it'll be safe. She shoots a fast backward glance at you as she disappears into the changing room.

Begin to grind your body against your partner's penis with more pressure. Push your bare breasts against his body, and move in any way that feels good to you and pleases him.

You climb out of the pool and look around for the lifeguard. You don't want him to see your hard-on. He's still occupied, so you slip into the family changing room unnoticed. As soon as you get around the corner, you see the woman standing and waiting for you. Without saying a word, she removes her bikini, first the top and then the bottom.

Slip out of your panties/bikini bottom. You can do this yourself under the covers, teasing him by taking your time, or you can have him help you.

She stands naked in front of you, shivering from the cold. You want nothing more than to caress her breasts and slip your cock into her trimmed pussy. You step toward her. She removes your bathing suit to free your erection. Eyeing your cock, she licks her lips. She sits down on one of the narrow wooden benches beside her, and then lies back, her legs straddling it.

If your partner is wearing pajamas or underwear, pull

them off. Then lie flat on your back with your arms over your head, and ask him to pull the covers off you to expose your naked body.

Continue to tell the story to give your partner a moment to enjoy your naked body in the sunlight.

You step over the bench with one leg so that the woman and the bench are between your legs. You bend your knees just a bit so that you're low enough to enter her. With one forceful motion, you bury your cock in her pussy. She lets out a grunt and pushes back against you. Lifting her arms over her head, she holds onto the bench for leverage. You start fucking her.

You fuck her slowly at first, savoring the sensation of your shaft sliding in and out of her pussy. You watch her body move as she squirms on the bench beneath you. Soon your body compels you to move faster. You fuck her faster. Her breasts begin dancing and you reach out to grab them, kneading them in your hands as she moves in pleasure below you. She opens her legs as wide as she can, pleading with you to go deeper.

Let your partner know that he can enter you at his leisure.

You fuck her hard and she loves it. She loves it so much that she starts coming all over your cock.

Let yourself come whenever you're ready, and then go back to the scene to bring your partner to orgasm.

Imagine yourself in this public changing room, fucking a woman you don't even know on a narrow, plastic bench. Her arms are over her head. She's clutching the bench for stability so that she can sustain the force of your thrusts. You're holding onto her breasts as your hips drive your cock deeper and deeper into her.

Have your partner put his hands on your breasts as he continues to thrust into you. If you can come again, do. If you can't, fake it if it helps bring your partner to orgasm. Just consider it part of the fantasy.

You feel her come again on your cock and her moans echo throughout the empty changing room. Someone could walk through the door at any moment. The thought of that makes you fuck her even harder . . . the threat of discovery is going to make you come so hard. You feel your orgasm building and soon you come violently inside her, squeezing her breasts and arching your back as the pleasure wracks your body.

Keep describing the scene to your partner until he comes.

Completely spent, you stand on weakened legs beside the bench, breathing heavily. You help the woman to her feet and she thanks you. You hand her a towel and she wraps it around herself, glowing. She smiles, and tells you that she hopes to see you again tomorrow morning. Swimming is the best exercise, she says, and she loved doing laps with you. She slips out of the changing room. You wait a few moments to avoid suspicion, then return to the pool and your regular morning workout.

AFTERWARD, tell your man how much you love being his swimming partner. Share a morning shower, and then make breakfast together. Expect to exchange a few smiles on the sly today, as memories of this morning's exercise routine pop into your minds. And remember that the smile on his face is for you, not for the early bird.

SEXY SNIPPETS

1. The woman is inches away from you in the empty pool. She's topless, and she pulls on her nipples to make them stick out and harden.

2. She floats on her back and spreads her legs open for you... you move her bikini bottom to the side.

3. She climbs out of the pool and heads into the changing room, looking behind herself to make sure you're following.

4. She squirms on the bench under you as you fuck her faster and faster, hoping nobody walks in on you.

5. You squeeze her breasts... she arches her back as you come powerfully inside her.

3

THE HYPNOTIST

*S*EX, SEX, SEX. It's all men think about, or so they say. Does the female mind have more discipline, or are women simply less obvious? Perhaps there are hundreds of women out there—going to work, getting groceries, standing in line at the bank—all of them thinking about sex. Perhaps some of them can't stop thinking about it. In this fantasy, your partner is a professional clinical hypnotist, whose assistance is being sought by a beautiful female client. She just can't seem to keep her mind from drifting toward the carnal even in the most inappropriate situations, and she needs his help to regain control of her wandering mind. At least that's what she claims.

This fantasy can be played out in bed, but you might want to play it out on the couch in the living room and pretend you're in the hypnotist's office. As with many of the other fantasies, begin this one by introducing an unexpected topic of conversation. Your partner spends most of his day talking to the same people about the same things. As his beloved, do your best to make him think about and discuss something other than the kids, the bills, the in-laws, or work.

You might say something to the effect of:

I heard today that men think about sex up to a hundred times a day. Do you think that's true? How do men get any work done?!

Sex and sexuality are always interesting topics to discuss, so don't race through the conversation to get to the physical part of the fantasy. Really engage your partner; get him actually trying to figure out how many times a day he thinks about sex. Ask him how many times sexual images flash across his mind, how many times he thinks about the two of you, and how many times in a day he might become aroused by sexual thoughts. Ask him when he typically has these thoughts, and if he ever has them at inappropriate times. Take your cues from him. If he seems amused by this conversation, keep it going. Talking about sex is linguistic foreplay.

Sooner or later, your partner will probably ask whether you think about sex during the day. Be truthful, but feel free to embellish a bit. If you want to learn about his sexuality and improve your sex life, the best way to earn his trust and get him to open up is to be open and honest yourself. Tell him of the times you have had sexual thoughts about him, and remember that there's nothing wrong with a little glorifying exaggeration! Flattery will get you everywhere. It will spice up the conversation, arouse him, and make him feel good about himself. And if he feels good about himself, he'll make you feel good.

When you're ready to set the scene for this fantasy, steer the conversation as follows:

I've heard that some people think about sex all the time. They're addicted to it... probably more men than women have that problem. Then again, there are a lot of promiscuous women out there, too. And probably a lot of women who just think about it but don't actually go through with it.

Slide into the storyline. Just as most of us enjoy an engaging conversation, so too do most of us love a good story. Again, don't rush through it. Sexual fantasies should offer more than just sex. They can be erotic short stories into which you and your partner can escape. Turn off the television tonight and use your imagination as entertainment.

Can you imagine some woman going through her day—going to work, shopping, driving the car, visiting friends, running errands—and all the while in the back of her mind she's thinking about sex? Everyone she looks at, she thinks of in a sexual way. She pictures almost everyone she sees without any clothes on. If she is looking at a man, her eyes inevitably wander to his groin; if she is looking at a woman, her eyes inevitably rest on her breasts or her ass. She tries to picture what it would be like to do something sexual to them, or for them to do something to her. She tries to put it out of her mind and concentrate on what she's doing, but she can't.

Take each of your partner's hands in turn, caressing and massaging them. Help him relax and get into the fantasy world. If you wish, move to the foot of the bed and massage each of his feet with small, but deep, strokes.

One day she's standing in line at the bank. She stares at the couples there together, and she starts to picture what they'd look like having sex... how they'd do it, whether she would suck on him, whether he would tongue her. She imagines everyone standing in line in an orgy. The sounds of grunting and groaning soon fill the bank, and people outside on the street stare through the windows to watch. She imagines the bank manager fucking the tellers one after the other in the vault. She's addicted to these thoughts, and they're beginning to rule and ruin her life.

The man in front of her strikes up an innocent conversation, and before she knows it, she's picturing his body on top of her, pinning her down. She can almost feel his weight press against her breasts, and his mouth press against her lips. She forgets what she's been saying to him, and finally he looks at her in a funny way, almost like he's clued in. She gets embarrassed and is relieved when it's his turn to approach the teller; he leaves, but within moments she's thinking about him again. She imagines the two of them undressing each other. She imagines him spreading her shirt open and cupping her breasts in his hands. She can almost feel her nipples harden and press against his palms.

Take your partner's hands, putting them first on your breasts, then moving them all over your body as the fantasy proceeds.

She imagines his hands moving down to caress her bare stomach, and then sliding cautiously between her legs... she opens her legs wider and he rubs her more boldly. The woman can feel herself getting wetter and wetter at the thought. Her breaths become deep and heavy, and her nipples start to tingle. She looks around the bank. Nobody is looking at her, nobody knows the dirty thoughts racing through her mind. Nobody knows how soaked her panties are getting. A teller becomes available and motions her over. She shakes her head and tries to stop the wave of arousal washing over her body, at least long enough to make the transaction. She can't wait to get back to her car, so she can drive to a secluded spot and masturbate.

She leaves the bank and drives to a quiet spot. She parks the car and hastily unzips her jeans, then fingers her clit until she comes with a shudder. Afterward, she decides that she has to do something about the sexual ideas and feelings that constantly intrude into her thoughts and overwhelm her will. She decides to seek the help of a hypnotist. She reasons that if they can help people stop smoking, they should be able to stop other types of addictions, including her addiction to sexual thoughts. She makes an appointment with a respected clinical hypnotist and waits in his office for him to appear. Even here and now she has to consciously ignore the sexual images flashing across her mind.

It's now time to let your partner know that you're in fantasy mode, if he hasn't realized it already. If you're in the living room, lie on the couch to pretend you're on the couch in the hypnotist's office, and have your partner sit close. If you're in bed, snuggle up close. Make sure he gets the message that you're in a playful, sexy mood. As always, be as descriptive as possible to help him visualize the fantasy world and its characters.

Say something like:

Imagine that you're a professional clinical hypnotist. You have a very respected practice. You see clients for a variety of reasons, everything from serious medical or psychological conditions to nail biting and smoking. You have an appointment with a new client, a woman, although you're not sure what her problem is. She wouldn't tell your secretary, she just said it was important. That's not too unusual, since some clients are em-

barrassed and don't want anyone other than you to know their reason for being there.

You walk into your office and notice a very attractive woman sitting on your black leather couch. She smiles nervously when you walk through the door, and she seems uneasy when you close it behind you. You sense that she is uncomfortable being alone with you, so you introduce yourself and shake hands. For a split second you think that her eyes focus on your groin, but you dismiss it. You sit across from her and engage in some small talk to loosen her up. She's very pretty and seems pleasant, although she is quite nervous.

Gently run your hands all over your partner's body. Don't just concentrate on the "hot zones" of his penis and testicles, but caress all parts of his body to physically stimulate him as much as possible.

You ask her why she needs to see you, and she says that she has a very embarrassing, very destructive addiction. After some assurances of confidentiality and gentle coaxing, the woman confesses that she has a sexual addiction. She is addicted to sexual thoughts . . . she explains that she has sexual thoughts about nearly everyone she sees. She says that she never acts on them—she's way too shy for that—but she's now masturbating fifteen or twenty times a day.

You tell her that you've seen this before, and that you're confident you can help. After she gives you permission to hypnotize her, you explain that, once she is under, you are going to explore her addiction, and then train her mind to overcome it. You ask her to lie back on the couch and relax. After only moments of your soothing voice, she becomes deeply hypnotized. You begin by asking her to describe a time when sexual thoughts overtook her.

Close your eyes as you tell the story with a sleepy voice; again, remember that erotic storytelling is effective foreplay.

The woman tells you that the most recent episode occurred only minutes ago. She tells you that while she was waiting for you in your office, she noticed a picture on your desk that she assumed, correctly, was of you. In the photo, you are holding some sort of plaque or award, and smiling. She tells you that she found you very handsome. She tells you that she felt a jolt of erotic electricity run through her body, warming her breasts and wetting her pussy, and that she knew her mind was going to wander.

You're a little taken aback, particularly since you find her quite attractive, but your professionalism kicks in and you distance yourself. She's a client, after all. You ask her to continue. She tells you that she started to imagine what would happen when you walked in the room and closed the door behind you. She tells you that she imagined lying back on the couch as you hypnotized her. After she was under your control, you came to sit beside her on the couch and unbuttoned her shirt. She imagined you staring at her breasts and slipping your fingers underneath the fabric of her bra to finger her nipples. She says she could feel her nipples get hard and her chest rise and fall under your exploring hands. She loved the feeling of being helplessly at the mercy of your desires.

You can take a break from your sexy storytelling to tease your man a little. Ask him if he's enjoying the story so far, and if he'd like you to continue. Ask him if he likes the feelings this fantasy is giving him. Enjoy his response. The realization that you are turning him on should arouse you even more.

She tells you that she imagined you would take advantage of her under hypnosis. She imagined that you would stand beside her so that your hips were close to her face, and that you would instruct her to reach over and unzip your pants. You would tell her to pull your cock out and lick it around the head. She pictured herself with your cock in her hands, flicking the head with her tongue, and sucking gently. Soon you would tell her to suck harder, and she would obey. She would feel the soft flesh of the head move past her lips until she felt the hardness of the shaft. She would suck gently, and then as hard as she could. She could picture her head bobbing up and down on your cock, and you rocking your hips back and forth, thrusting yourself into her mouth.

Despite your professionalism, her descriptions quicken your breathing and make you hard. You're struck that she is completely under hypnosis and that you could do whatever you want to her. You could stand up right now and within seconds have your cock plunging in and out of her mouth. She wouldn't know the difference between relaying her imaginings and the real thing. And she wouldn't remember a thing . . . you could make sure of it. You look at her, and again notice how beautiful she is. Her lips are red and full, and they'd feel exquisite wrapped tightly around your hardening rod. You glance at the door. It's locked. You're safe.

Concentrate your caresses on your partner's penis and testicles while you are describing this hypnotic blow job.

Continue with the fantasy, but now begin to actually perform what you are describing.

You know the woman is deep under hypnosis. You tell her that you're going to give her a set of instructions that she will obey, but that she will completely forget upon waking. You have no intention of really violating her, but you're aroused and you decide there's no harm in just watching her. In fact, you reason that it might even be therapeutic for her to act out some of her addictive behavior. You instruct her to demonstrate how she normally masturbates. In dutiful response, her hips start to gyrate and lift off the couch.

Move your body likewise.

Keeping her eyes closed, she reaches between her legs and briefly rubs herself, arching her back and beginning to moan in pleasure. Next, she unbuttons her shirt to reveal full breasts covered by a red bra made of very thin, almost see-through material. You can clearly make out her hard nipples poking through the fabric. She reaches behind herself and unsnaps her bra, allowing the soft mounds of her breasts to come free. Her nipples harden when they are exposed to the room air, and you gaze at them, erect and pink in the center of her generous breasts.

Without standing up, she unzips her pants and squirms out of them, throwing them to the floor. She is so passionate, so turned on, that you can see she has soaked through her pink panties. Her body is writhing and sliding along the couch. She lifts her hips up, straining to find a body to push against... straining to find a hard cock to sink into her pussy. She takes off her panties to reveal a neatly trimmed pussy swollen with excitement. You're struck with the image of your cock buried into it, but you try to put it out of your head.

Remove your clothing as sensually as you can, enjoying the fact that your partner is watching you with bated breath. Immerse yourself in your role. Imagine you are free of all inhibitions, and that you are masturbating in this man's office while he watches with mounting desire for you. Move your body as if you are being ravished by some invisible Apollo, and make throaty sounds of your pleasure.

The woman starts to moan and groan louder but you tell her to remain quiet. You don't want your secretary hearing anything strange from your office. You watch as she silently stimulates her body further. With outstretched fingers, she moves her hands all over her naked breasts and stomach, and slips them between her legs to finger her pussy. When she pulls them out, they're glistening. With wet fingers, she pinches and tweaks her nipples, making them even harder.

At this point in the fantasy, you may wish to ask your partner what he would do to this woman if he were the hypnotist, and then act out his ideas. Would he make her come by masturbating? Would he make her walk around the room naked? Would he make her suck on him? How would he have sex with her? If he wishes, your partner can determine how this fantasy ends. (If you are not comfortable with the element of unawareness in this fantasy, imagine instead that the woman is feigning hypnosis to satisfy her own sexual desires.)

Or you can continue with the prescribed fantasy, as follows:

Against all ethics, you stand up and step toward her until your hips are close to her face. It's not enough to just watch her anymore. You're overcome with erotic desire from watching her touch herself, and from staring at her lustful, voluptuous naked body. You reach down and trace a nipple with a finger, and you realize that the nipple is almost as hard as your cock.

You tell the woman to act out her sexual thoughts. Without hesitation, she reaches over and unzips your pants. She pushes them and your boxers down to your ankles, takes your cock in her hands, and begins to gently lick the head. She moves her soft, warm tongue across it, and then pushes it through tightly pursed lips, into her mouth. The skin on the head is stretched back as she forces it through the resistance of her lips, and you get rock-hard in response. You tell her to suck harder and she obeys.

You can feel the strong pull of her suck draw your cock force-fully into her mouth, and you can feel her moist lips pass tightly over your shaft. Suddenly she places her hands on your ass and drives your dick deeper and harder into her mouth. You arch your back and stare at the ceiling, abandoning yourself to the pulsing and pulling sensations in your cock and balls.

You can be performing oral sex in any position; just ensure that you take enough breathers to remind your man where he is and what he is doing in the fantasy world. You can be performing oral sex on him while he is standing beside you on the bed or the couch, while he is lying flat on his back, while he is kneeling above you, or while he is resting on his knees and leaning back on his arms.

Then return to the fantasy.

Imagine your cock being sucked by this woman ... she's completely hypnotized, unaware of what you're making her do. When she wakes up, she won't remember a thing. She won't remember that she was clutching your ass and swallowing your shaft as far as she could down her throat. She seemed very conservative when you met her, and despite her sexual addiction, she would never have really chosen to do this. But here she is, giving a blow job to a total stranger. Her breasts are exposed and her nipples are taut, and her pussy is dripping.

Continue to move your body as if it is overcome by sexual ecstasy. Arch your back, throw your head around, sigh heavily, rock and gyrate your hips, and thrust your breasts into the air. Get into it. Sexual enthusiasm is contagious, and the more passionate you are, the more your partner will respond in kind.

Both her body and yours are in an extreme state of sexual excitement. You know that an orgasm is building, and you think about how you want to come. In her mouth or in her pussy? Do you want to shoot your come down her throat, or do you want to grind your hips against her pussy and shoot your come into it? All traces of your detached professionalism are gone ... now you're just a man who needs to get off. You need to feel that release explode from your body into hers.

At this point in the fantasy, you should determine how you and your partner want to experience your orgasms. We will provide two alternate endings that you and your partner may enjoy.

If your man wants to come in your mouth, continue as follows:

You tell the woman to suck on your dick again and this time not to stop until she feels you come in her mouth. She curls her fingers tightly around the base of your shaft, wraps her lips around the head, and then pushes her mouth down to swallow the entire length of your cock. You surrender completely to the pounding pleasure between your legs as your shaft disappears into her mouth. She squeezes your balls gently but firmly until they ache with pleasure and threaten to explode.

Perform oral sex on your partner until he comes in your mouth. He will enjoy the thought and sensation of your lips around him while he ejaculates, but as with the other fantasies that involve oral sex, it's up to you whether you swallow. If they are being brutally honest, many men will admit that the sexual heaven of a blow job is perfected when the woman follows through all the way, and swallows. However, oral sex is so enjoyable that it doesn't really matter, and if you find the idea uncomfortable, don't do it.

Continue to break intermittently to allow yourself to finish describing the rest of the fantasy. While you talk, continue to stimulate him, tracing his body with your fingers, cupping his balls and stroking his penis.

You can feel your orgasm building and you reach down to grab the woman's head. You shove it into your groin and she wildly sucks your rigid cock. She can't wait to taste the come in her mouth. You tell her that you want her to swallow it. You don't want to see a drop on her lips, you want her to swallow it all. Without any warning, her whole body shakes violently and your realize that she has experienced a very strong orgasm in her sleeplike state.

If you wish, you can ask your man to use his fingers on you while you are sucking on him, and to bring you to orgasm that way.

Her orgasm brings you close to coming yourself, especially as you realize that soon she'll be sitting across from you, oblivious to what just went on. Suddenly, your orgasm peaks and your rod pulses as waves of come stream into the woman's mouth. You feel an incredible, consuming wave of pleasure, and keep grinding your public hair against her mouth until the last drop is squeezed out of your cock, and your orgasm ebbs away.

If instead you or your man want to come during sexual intercourse, continue as follows:

You tell the woman you want to drive your hard cock into her. You tell her to spread her legs as wide as she can, and let you in... you're going to fuck her, and you know she's going to like it. She spreads her legs and you see the pink folds of her slippery pussy spread apart just slightly, in anticipation of you. You climb on top of her on the couch and in one fast, decisive stroke, you fill her with your hardness. You feel the head of your cock sink deep into her warm, tight flesh, and you feel the lips of her pussy wrap around your shaft. Your whole length disappears into her body. She opens her legs even wider and pushes herself against you, grinding her wetness against your pubic hair.

Invite your partner to climb on top of you and penetrate you. Continue to lead him through the fantasy as he thrusts, and until both of you have reached orgasm.

You start fucking the woman. You pull your entire length out of her, and then plunge it back in again. Again and again you pound this woman, fucking her fast and hard. She has a cock inside her and she loves it. One of her fantasies is coming true, and she doesn't even know it. Without any warning, her whole body shakes violently and your realize that she has experienced a very strong orgasm in her sleeplike state. Her orgasm brings you close to coming yourself. Soon she'll be sitting across from you, oblivious to what just went on, thinking that the wetness between her legs is only her own juices, not a strange man's come.

You feel your orgasm building. Your cock is so swollen and so hard, and your balls are aching for release. With one arm you reach under the woman's ass and lift it up toward you, allowing you to thrust even deeper. Suddenly, your orgasm peaks and your rod pulses as waves of come stream into the woman's pussy. You feel an incredible, consuming wave of pleasure, and keep grinding your pubic hair against her crotch until the last drop is squeezed out of your cock, and your orgasm ebbs away.

However you and your partner have decided to come, conclude the fantasy as follows:

You pull yourself away from the woman and clean yourself off in your office bathroom. You bring a wet cloth and clean the woman off before instructing her to dress herself again. As you wake her, you tell her she won't remember a thing, but she'll feel a strong sense of well-being. After she's awake, you recommend that she visit you monthly, just to ensure the addiction is kept in check. She happily agrees. As she leaves your office, she flashes you a mischievous, knowing grin over her shoulder.

AFTERWARD, tell your partner what a great time you had leading him through this fantasy. Reassure him that you will never need to be in a state of altered awareness to find him irresistible. Tell him how wonderful his penis looks and feels, and how well he uses it. Tell him you love how his hardness feels in your mouth, and how his incredible size fills you up inside. Tell him what he wants to hear. If he wants to drift off to sleep, let him. And, as always, remember that the smile on his face is for you, not for the sleepy sex addict.

Sexy Snippets

1. *She's lying hypnotized on the couch, describing her fantasy of being taken advantage of by you.*
2. *You can touch her anywhere, and tell her to do anything... she won't remember a thing.*
3. *She starts to moan louder, but you tell her to keep quiet— you don't want your secretary to hear anything.*
4. *With sleeping eyes, she clutches your ass and drives your cock deeper into her mouth.*
5. *You're fucking her fast on the couch... her fantasy is coming true, and she doesn't even know it.*

4

THE NAUGHTY BABYSITTER

*O*UR PARTNERS may be fairly conservative, strait-laced men with predictable lives. They go to work, come home, and occasionally take us out on the town. That doesn't mean they conform sexually, though. The idea of an older, married man and a young babysitter alone in a car together quickly arouses many men. It is the strong social taboo against seducing young women that makes it perfect material for an exciting fantasy.

The great thing about this love scene is that you can play it out in your bedroom just by whispering it in your partner's ear; or, for a completely unexpected thrill, you can play it out in the car. Sex *and* cars? Two of your partner's favorite things together at last. In this fantasy, your partner gets far more than a half-hearted thank-you and a slammed door when he drives the babysitter home.

If you choose to act out this fantasy in the car, pick a

night when your partner and you are driving home from an evening out and find a way to bring up the subject of babysitters. If you have one waiting for your return at home, you might say something like:

I hope the kids behaved for So-and-so.

If you don't have kids, you can fabricate something like:

So-and-so at work was telling me about her babysitter... she ran up her long-distance phone bill last weekend.

After a moment of silent but staged reflection, you might mischievously ask:

Honey, you know the cliché of the married man and the young babysitter? I wonder how often it happens? I mean, when he's driving her home at night and they're alone together in a dark car, sitting so close, do you think either one of them thinks about it? Everyone knows how taboo it is.

Set the scene for your man while you touch his arm, or maybe his thigh.

Do you think you'd get turned on? If you were alone in the car at night with the young babysitter, driving her home, do you think your mind would wander? Imagine that the streets are empty, there's hardly any traffic at this hour. I'm waiting for you at home, and not suspecting a thing. Meanwhile, this girl is sitting right beside you, so close that your legs are touching.

Tease your partner playfully to let him know it's okay for him to think about this with you. You could laugh, touch his hair, or trace the outline of his ear with your finger.

Imagine that she's the same babysitter we've used for years, since she was barely a teenager. But you've noticed lately that she's grown up... she's in college now, and you don't remember ever seeing evidence of breasts under her shirt before. We're

*friends with her parents, and lately her dad has been com-
plaining a lot about her behavior. He's told us that he knows
she's out with boys a lot. You suspect he knows she's not a virgin
anymore. After all, the last couple times you've driven her home
it almost seemed like she was flirting with you.*

Sketch the details that let your partner effortlessly visualize his fantasy world. Continue to touch him, moving closer
if you can, putting both your hands on his body and leaning
in close so your breasts graze his arm. Breathe into his ear or
nibble his earlobe while you tell the story.

*What would you do if you were driving down a dark, quiet
street toward her house? You're almost there when she starts
telling you about the boy she's dating. She starts going on about
how the boys her age don't know what they're doing when it
comes to sex. You're caught completely off guard by her can-
dor... she's never spoken like this before to you. She rests her
hand on the inside of your thigh, and instantly you feel a rush.
Your pants feel tighter.*

Slide a little closer to your partner, and begin caressing his
inner thigh, working your way closer and closer to his groin.

*She tells you that she's been fantasizing about being with an
older, experienced man... she admits she lost her virginity to a
boy her own age, so there's nothing for her to lose now. She says
the boy didn't seem very good at what he was doing, and she
isn't even sure that he did it right. She wants to try a real man
now. She turns her head and stares at you, enjoying the uncomfortable effect her frankness and physical closeness are having
on you.*

Pause. Stare at your partner teasingly and bite your lip.
Run your hands through your hair, maybe girlishly curling a
strand around your finger.

When her house is in view, she casually mentions that she'd like to spend a little more time talking with you before you take her home. She suggests that you find a secluded spot where the two of you can spend a few minutes together. What do you do? Do you drive her home and walk her to her door? No. I think you don't respond, but you drive past her house and search for a safe place to park the car. You don't know why you didn't stop at her house. You don't know why you're doing something as insane as this. You both know that you're not interested in talking.

You find a quiet, dark spot, and you pull into it, flicking off the headlights. You cut the engine and an awkward, sexually tense silence fills the interior of the car. You sit and wait for her to take the lead before you might have to. You don't have to wait long. The next thing you know, she promises that she won't tell her dad—or me.

Tell your partner to find a quiet, hidden place to park the car. Tell him to hurry so he'll know you're excited. After you've found a good spot, continue the fantasy.

Then her hands are on you, and she unzips your pants. You push yourself against the back of the seat as she frees the head of your cock. Without a moment's hesitation, she puts her head in your lap and begins sucking you. The sudden and unexpected sensation sends the blood racing to your groin and you clench the steering wheel. Your cock throbs as her lips pass over the head and her mouth swallows the shaft. You can feel it against the back of her throat.

With this, lean into your man's groin and begin to suck and stroke his penis as though it were the most delicious thing you've ever had in your mouth. But only for a few moments. Then coax him into the backseat, where the real action is going to happen.

She stops sucking on you, and without missing a beat she crawls into the backseat and tells you to follow. Again she promises you that nobody will know, she wants to keep it as secret as you do. She tells you to hurry, since if you take too long I'll be wondering where you are or if something happened to you. I'd never suspect that you're climbing into the backseat with the babysitter. I don't know anything about this part of you, and would never believe it anyway.

You can't believe you're doing this, but without even thinking about it you do what she says and climb into the backseat with her. As soon as you're there, she pulls off her shirt in one quick motion and lies flat on her back on the seat. She draws her legs up and with bent knees, spreads them open. She asks you to unzip her jeans and pull them down. Things are happening so fast that you can't even process them. You can tell she's done this before, and you wonder if any of your friends who use her as a babysitter have had her like this.

At this point, you should be lying on the backseat as you have described the babysitter doing, with your shirt off and your legs open. Delight in the feeling of having yourself exposed in this way. And get into the role! Really pretend that you're this young, relatively inexperienced girl who is offering herself to an older, sexually skilled man. You'll love anticipating what's next.

The muffled sounds of the interior of the car, the cramped space, the unfamiliar feeling of the car seat against bare skin, the unknown location, and the darkness will all serve to heighten the realism of this forbidden fantasy. If you are just whispering this fantasy in his ear, be sure to describe the setting in vivid detail so both of you can feel the excitement.

It's a really tight space back there, but you don't notice. In fact, it adds to the excitement. You notice the windows have steamed up, and for a second you hope that I won't notice when you pull up in our driveway. But the thought passes, and you look down at the girl underneath you.

She's stretched out with her arms over her head, elbows bent. She's wearing a little black bra with tiny roses on it. Her breasts are small but you feel an incredible urge to pull off her bra and see them naked. You reach down and touch the zipper on her jeans, and the moment you do, your cock stiffens even more than before. You pull the zipper down and it separates to reveal her pubic hair. She isn't wearing any panties, and her pubic hair is shaved and shaped into a little heart.

You too should be panty-free. If your partner isn't already straining at the gate like a mad racehorse, this unexpected sight will set him off.

You struggle to pull her jeans down past her knees, and once they're down you pull your own pants down. You don't need the rest of your clothes off, you just need your cock free.

Unless your man wants it otherwise, let him enjoy this fantasy with you more undressed than he is.

The girl is arching her back and wriggling in anticipation. You reach down and feel her pubic hair, slipping your thumb down to feel her. She's very slippery. You spread her legs open more and climb on top of her. You're only a split second away from penetrating her. Even if you could stop yourself at this point, you've come so far that it doesn't matter.

She tells you to wait one second. She says, "Please, please suck my nipples first." She really likes that. She struggles to put her hands under her back and unfastens her bra. She lets it drop to the floor and for the first time you see her breasts completely exposed. They're small, almost flat, but incredibly sexy.

You bend over her and take one of her pink nipples in your mouth. It's as hard as a rock. You suck it as hard as you can and bite at it. She lets out a loud groan that takes you by surprise and makes your balls throb. She grabs both her breasts in her hands, and sticks them out for you. She tells you to suck them as hard as you can, don't worry about hurting her. She likes them sucked really hard, and the guys she knows don't do it right. You suck them as hard as you can, wanting to satisfy her so she'll let you come inside.

If you would rather your partner do something else than suck your nipples, simply substitute what you prefer in the fantasy. Such is the bonus of being the storyteller!

Allow your partner to get as physical as he wants, to immerse you and him in the fantasy world more completely. And make lots of noise. The sound of sex is an incredibly effective aphrodisiac. Accordingly, alter the tone and quality of your voice as much as possible to help your partner imagine that the moans, grunts, and sighs are coming from this girl, not from his familiar partner. Also, change the way you normally move your body. Clutch, grab, squirm, and do everything possible to help him imagine there is a new and different body underneath him. Lose yourself in your desperation for him. Act like a sex-crazed teenager and enjoy the freedom.

Finally, she pushes your head away from her breasts and tells you to do it. She whispers to you that she's never had an orgasm before, but that she knows you can make her experience one. Without a moment's hesitation you grab onto your cock and position it at the slit of her pussy. You plunge it in with one fast stroke and feel it sink into her hot tightness.

As your partner nears orgasm, tell him how good he is and

how crazy he is making you. In this fantasy, he is the experienced, sexually skilled older man, so make him feel that way.

You're thrusting fast and hard because you just want to get off as fast as you can. The girl wraps her legs around your back and squeezes your body tightly. She's trying to lift her pelvis and her pussy so you can plunge even deeper inside her. You keep pounding her as hard and as fast as you can. You look at her face and her mouth is open, moans of pleasure coming out of it. She is having her first orgasm. She groans and tells you how well you use your cock. She wants you to fill her up. You're fucking her so hard the whole car is shaking, and she has to brace herself against the car door. Your orgasm is building, and finally you come inside her.

It shouldn't take long before you both reach orgasm, and your partner collapses on top of you, completely drained and satisfied.

As the pleasure ebbs, you collapse on top of her. She tells you, "That's what I've been waiting for." You collect yourselves, and then you weakly climb behind the wheel. You drive to her house in silence, and she gives you a quick kiss on the cheek when you arrive. With a sly wink, she jumps out of the car and sprints to the front door.

On a basic housekeeping note, be sure to have placed something within reach to clean yourselves up before driving home. Always be prepared for the aftermath.

AFTERWARD, enjoy the drive home and share a laugh about your little detour. Tell your partner what your regular hourly babysitting rate is, but that tonight you'll take a drive-thru cheeseburger or ice cream cone in lieu of it. Food tastes better than ever after sex, so indulge yourselves. Make sure to tell your partner how good he made you feel, and what an exceptional lover he is. Tell him how wonderful it feels to have him inside you, and how much fun you always have with him. And remember that the smile on his face as he glows behind the wheel is for you, not for the boisterous babysitter.

Sexy Snippets

1. *You're in the front seat of the car…the babysitter unzips your pants and quickly begins to give you head.*

2. *She wants you so badly. She knows you can use your cock to make her have her first orgasm, since the boys her age couldn't.*

3. *She struggles to put her hands under her back to unfasten her bra. Her breasts are small, almost flat, but incredibly sexy.*

4. *She's moving and groaning in your backseat, lost in how you feel and how skilled you are.*

5. *She tells you to drive it in her harder and harder. You're so good at it, and she tells you nobody will ever know about the two of you.*

5

THE HOLE IN THE WALL

ANONYMITY can bring a thrill to the sexual experience. In this fantasy, you will allow your partner to revel in raw, anonymous sex. He will love the idea of being the gluttonous recipient of paid pleasure, without having to return the favor—at least not tonight. This fantasy compounds the thrill of anonymity with a raunchiness that will make any respiring man breathe heavier. It gets right to the point and stays there.

This fantasy is a great one if you're not necessarily in the mood for intercourse, but still wish to pleasure your partner. It's certainly not a fantasy you will choose if you're in the mood for a long evening of lovemaking, since it features fellatio exclusively. If you're not in the habit of performing oral sex on your man, you may not be entirely comfortable with it. But if you're willing to give it a try, you may find that you enjoy it as much as he does.

This fantasy begins before you crawl into bed. Whether you're watching television before turning in or engaged in your nighttime routine, find a way to bring up the topic.

You can fabricate something like this:

I was channel surfing tonight and there was a show on about those sex clubs... those places are pretty raunchy, you know. They were showing some of what goes on in them. Have you ever been to one?

We promise your partner will be interested in learning more and will prompt you to elaborate. When you've aroused his curiosity, playfully lead him into your dark bedroom. Keep him standing.

Begin to undress your partner with a mischievous smile while you tell him about what you saw going on inside the sex club.

They had this one room that you wouldn't believe. It was all dark and dirty, and you could hear the pounding of the loud music from the main part of the club. These men were lined up facing a wall, and they were completely naked. They were standing very close to the wall with their chests pressed against it. You could see that at waist level there were holes in the wall.

Go slowly and let him get a good picture of this in his mind. Undress him completely so that he is standing naked in your bedroom with you standing in front of him. Keep talking while you undress him, brushing your fingers against his skin and kissing his belly or thighs. Then continue with the scene.

Can you picture yourself standing in front of a wall like that? You're very aware of your nakedness, and of the fact that all these strangers are in the same position as you. There are dividers between the men, and they offer just enough privacy so that you can relax. You're in the basement of some sex club and it doesn't get any dirtier than this.

Imagine that you're standing with your chest against this wall. All of a sudden you experience a wave of sensation as fingers touch and then wrap around your cock. You look down and see a woman's hand with dark red nail polish pulling it through the hole in the wall. You get hard really fast, so she has a lot to hold on to. You have absolutely no idea what she looks like or what's behind the wall. All you know is that you're on this side of the wall but your aching dick is on the other side, at the mercy of this woman's hands.

At this point you should be holding on to your partner's penis lightly. Get onto your knees in front of him and very softly run your fingertips over the shaft of his penis. Apply only enough pressure to get him hard.

It feels like every drop of blood in your body is pulsating to your cock and balls. It feels like every nerve in your body is localized between your legs, and you can't feel any other part of your body. Your entire consciousness is focused on your groin.

You want him to think of and feel nothing but the sensations stirring in his groin.

You're frozen, pressing the front of your body against the wall, and waiting to see what she'll do to you. You look down but can't see your cock or her fingers anymore, they're on the other side of the wall. You can feel the woman's hands caressing the shaft, just teasing it with her fingertips. You're getting harder by the second. In the back of your mind you're hoping that you'll feel her wet lips wrap around it.

With one motion, lick the underside of your partner's penis from the base of his shaft to the head. When you get to the tip, purse your lips and gently kiss and suck it. Flick your tongue all around the head of the penis and the frenulum. Suck and lick the head at the same time, and stretch the skin on top of the head by pushing it back with your lips. Swallow as much of his shaft as you can, but only do this once before again concentrating on the head.

Add a hand job by moving your hand up and down the shaft. You can use your whole hand, or just your index finger and thumb in an "O." Make sure that your hand is wet (lick it if there isn't enough saliva from your mouth) and that you are alternating your speed and pressure. Go slow and steady, then lightly and quickly. Don't let your partner get too accustomed to any one rhythm or sensation this early on—save that for when he is building momentum for his orgasm.

Stop using your hand. Flick your tongue, lick, and kiss along the length of his shaft. Bury your face in the pubic hair at the base. Reach under his scrotum to gently squeeze and fondle his testicles. Suck them, lick them, and move them around in your hand. Start stroking his shaft again, using both hands in any way that you like. Make twisting and pulling motions as you move your hands up and down.

Carefully observe your partner's reactions to what you are doing. If he likes something, repeat it. If he starts to soften, stop whatever you're doing and try something else. Your ability to speak to him during this fantasy will obviously be compromised by now, but he won't mind! Still, take a moment every now and then, when you are only using your hands, to refresh his visualization and describe what is happening to him.

You can't believe this is happening to you like this... it's so dirty, and all you can feel is your cock being sucked expertly by someone you can't even see.

Remember to moan and make other sounds of enjoyment to arouse you and your partner even more while you have him in your mouth. By now he will be ready and anxious for you to adopt a stronger and more rhythmic pace to your blow/hand job. Purse your lips tightly before you slide the head of his penis past them and into your mouth; this slight resistance and release will feel heavenly.

Squeeze your hand or fingers harder as you move up and down the shaft of your man's penis. Squeeze his testicles with more urgency, but not necessarily with more pressure. Suck and lick at the same time while moving your mouth up and down, past the head and along the shaft. Suck hard as you pull your mouth off of his penis. Find a pace and rhythm that will allow him to build the momentum he needs to orgasm.

Let your partner know it's okay for him to come in your mouth whenever he wants to. After he comes, keep stroking with your hand until he tells you to stop. The head of the penis will still be sensitive, so let the aftereffects of his orgasm linger as long as possible.

AFTERWARD, make sure to tell your partner how much you enjoyed doing that to him, and how good he feels in your mouth. Enjoy his release and relaxation with him. And remember that the smile on his face as he drifts off to sleep is for you, not for the faceless woman on the other side of the wall.

6

PLAYING DOCTOR

*T*HE NAME of this fantasy speaks for itself, but in this book the children's game is all grown up. In this role-play, you will create sexual tension out of the sense of exposure and surrender that is a part of doctor-patient interaction. You will guide your partner through a fantasy in which he is an unethical doctor, about to take sexual advantage of a vulnerable female patient. But fear not—the outcome is mutual pleasure, not malpractice.

When you're lying in bed with your partner and chatting, catch his attention by telling him the following:

I don't remember where I first heard this, but did you know that doctors used to perform vaginal massages on their female patients? People thought that hysteria could be cured, or at least calmed, if the woman received a vaginal massage. Can you believe that? I can't believe doctors would ever buy into that. It makes you wonder if they really believed it, or they just used it as an excuse to get off on their female patients. Maybe they just liked the fact that they could make a woman come like that.

If your partner is genuinely amused by this discussion, keep it going. You'll get to the physical part of the fantasy soon enough, so slow down and let yourselves enjoy the process.

Touch your partner with soft, sweet caresses while you talk. Cuddle up to him or trace along his skin with your fingertips. Draw attention to your body by playing with your hair or otherwise touching yourself.

I mean, just picture this poor woman going in for an examination, and the next thing she knows, she's lying naked on the examining table, feeling completely exposed and wondering what's going to happen to her.

Smile while you're telling the story, and offer playful hints to your partner to let him know you want him to think about this.

Can you picture that? Do you think when she climbed onto the table the doctor thought about what he was going to do? Do you think that as he was looking at her naked body, trembling and waiting for his hands to touch her, he thought about making her have an orgasm under cover of an examination? I mean, he's a doctor, so he knows all about a woman's body ... he could pretend to be examining her vagina, but really be trying to see if he could make her have an orgasm. He knows she's very modest and shy, and won't want to show that it feels good.

Mischievously tell your man that you'd like to pretend you're getting a vaginal massage. And what woman wouldn't? This fantasy is highly erotic for both men and women; he will enjoy the sense of sexual control, while you'll enjoy the opportunity to be touched exactly how you want to be touched.

This fantasy has the added bonus of being a great teacher—while your partner is "massaging" your body, you can show him what arouses you the most.

Would you do something for me? Would you pretend that you're the doctor and I'm that patient?

Remove your clothes, lie flat on your back on the bed, and have your partner kneel beside you. You're going to talk him through this examination and this fantasy by instructing him to perform what you describe.

Imagine that she's lying naked on the examining table, and you come over beside her. You tell her you're going to examine her breasts first, and you begin to feel them. You start under the arms, then move your fingers in a circular motion all around each breast, to the nipple. When you get to the nipple, you rub it between your fingers, and pinch it a little. You tell her you're checking to see if it responds properly to stimuli.

While your partner is touching you, respond with pleasure when he does something you like, but don't hesitate to help him out. It won't break fantasy mode if you gently guide his hands on your breasts. Take the opportunity to have him caress you exactly how you like.

She's had breast exams in the past, but they've never felt like this before. She can't quite put her finger on what is different this time. It's almost like your hands are moving too slowly, too deliberately. Although this is a medical exam, she can't help but feel her nipples respond in an almost sexual way. You can feel them harden under your fingers, and you know she's embarrassed, but aroused. She's hoping you don't notice, but she knows you do. She's hoping that she won't betray her feelings. She'd be mortified if the doctor thought she was turned on by his examining her breasts.

You keep kneading her breasts and rubbing and pinching her nipples. She feels an incredible urge to respond by arching her back. She has to force herself to press her back into the table to prevent it from arching to meet your touch. She tries to distract herself by looking at the posters and calendar on the wall. Still, she can't fight the feeling that something isn't quite right. That you're taking a little too long to do this, and that you're touching her differently than last time. She can't quite identify what is different, but it's beginning to feel wrong. You finish the exam, and when you take your hands away she feels a slight ache as her breasts miss your touch.

Have your man stop touching your breasts, and tell him you want to feel his fingers between your legs.

You tell her that you're going to do the vaginal exam now, and you move toward her feet. You bend her knees and position yourself between her legs.

Have him position himself similarly.

She feels a rush of exposure as the cool room air hits her vagina. She looks down and sees you looking at her pussy. She couldn't be more exposed or vulnerable than she is right now. She still feels a strange tingling sensation from the breast massage, and she's afraid that she may be a little wet down there from it. She's hoping against hope that she's not, or that you won't notice. You take a sheet and place it over her knees. It covers the front of her thighs so she can no longer see what you're doing down there.

There is an element of unawareness in this fantasy that is similar to that in the hypnotist fantasy. Again, if you are uncomfortable with this aspect, omit it. Rather than making the patient innocent and unaware, you can make her experienced and strategic. You can have her specifically request a vaginal massage from the doctor for "therapeutic" reasons, and then instruct him on what pleasures a woman. But don't be ashamed if the woman's vulnerability and unknowingness turn you on. Our fantasies are not always politically correct.

In accordance with the fantasy, place the bedsheets over your knees so you cannot directly see what your partner is doing.

She holds her breath and waits for you to touch her between her legs. She's determined for it not to feel good. Finally she feels your fingers pressing against the lips of her vagina. They're slippery from the lubricating jelly. You gently insert the tip of a finger into her pussy. You tell her that she's very tense and tight, and that she must be stressed out. But you know that's nonsense. You tell her that you're going to try a new technique on her. It's worked wonders for other women.

You tell her that you're going to massage her vagina at the same time that you're examining it. She feels your finger slide farther into her. She feels you move it around inside her, circling and pressing. You can see the blood drain from her face in response. You're exploring inside her body with your finger, and obviously she's not used to being touched in those places. She holds as still as possible. She's terrified that it's going to feel good.

Just as you did during the "breast exam," instruct your partner on how best to touch you. Take his fingers and move them where you like, or tell him what feels good.

Soon you begin to make her fears come true. Her pussy begins to ache and throb. It's wet down there, she can feel it, but she's hoping it's from the lubricating jelly. But she knows it's her, and she's praying you can't tell the difference. You begin to push your finger in, and then pull it out. You're imitating sex, and that has an effect on her body. You can tell she's fighting the urge to rock her hips in response. You keep doing it, each time pushing your finger in farther.

Suddenly you stop and pull your finger out. Her body aches to feel that sensation again, no matter how wrong it is. She looks down and you know she's watching you look at her pussy. You have no expression on your face. You know she's trying to convince herself that this must be just a regular examination, but it's beginning to feel so strongly sexual that she doesn't trust herself.

Since you are being touched precisely how you like, you shouldn't have any trouble showing your man how aroused you are. Tell him to touch your clitoris, or move his fingers in a specific way—show him what feels good.

Without warning, you touch her clitoris and begin to stimulate it. She steadies herself by pushing her feet into the stirrups. You can see her clitoris is swelling. You keep stroking it. Involuntarily she tightens her lower body. Your cock is throbbing hard with desire for her. She's ready now. She's ready to take your cock in her pussy, although she'll never really know it was there. Her body begins to wriggle and move underneath you. She can't stop it. It feels so good, it's completely out of her control. You tell her that you need to move a little closer to get a better angle. She doesn't respond, too afraid that her voice will come out as a moan and betray her weakness.

Indicate that you want your partner to penetrate you, unless you want to come with him just touching you. Let him see how much his perfect caresses have turned you on. You can bet he'll remember what pleases you.

This time when your finger goes inside her, it feels different.

It's thicker, especially at the tip. She looks down at you, and you are closer to her body. She can't tell for sure, but it's almost like your body is moving ever so slightly back and forth. The thought pops into her mind that you've stuck your penis inside her, but she dismisses the idea immediately. You look down to see what she can't. Your cock is plunging deep inside her. Her soft pink folds of skin are wrapped tightly around your shaft, and they grip it as you slide it in and out of her body. She's being fucked and she doesn't even know it. You're fucking her and it feels wonderful.

Allow yourself to get lost in the fantasy. Your man has touched you exactly how you like, and now he's inside you, pleasuring you even more. Imagine that you're struggling to fight off the pleasure, but the feeling is just too wonderful to resist.

There's no way, she tells herself. It just feels different. You start to thrust your cock inside her faster and harder.

As you and your partner make love, keep the fantasy alive by whispering in his ear, as follows:

Imagine you're this doctor who everyone thinks is so up-standing. You're in a small examination room with this naked woman lying before you on the table. She's yours. You can do things to her body and make her experience sensations that she can't fight. You know she's having sexual feelings and that she's trying to fight them. You know she can't say anything, since she isn't sure if this is really happening or not. You know she's close to coming.

When you look down, you can see your smooth, glistening shaft moving in and out of her. She thinks it's your finger. She can't see what's going on behind the sheet on her knees. You know she's wildly excited but is trying hard to fight it. You struggle to remain expressionless. She's confused by what she's feeling, but your face doesn't betray your feelings or your mounting orgasm.

Allow yourself to come while still imagining yourself in the fantasy situation.

A warmth washes over her entire body, and despite trying as hard as she can to stop it, she can feel an orgasm building. She's humiliated, but so turned on that she can't stop it. Right now she'd rather face humiliation than have you stop what you're doing. You knew you could bring her to this point. She does her best not to move too much, only enough to meet your thrusts. They come harder and harder until her orgasm peaks and she comes, sending a visible shudder throughout her body.

Now it's your partner's turn. Tell him you want to feel him come too.

You know that your own orgasm is building. Almost unexpectedly, your cock shoots come into her pussy and you feel the release in your groin. She feels a gush of hot liquid inside her, and for a moment she thinks that a groan escapes your lips.

Let him come inside you.

You stop thrusting, pull your cock out, and wipe her off with a towel. You tell her that her exam is over and that she can get dressed. She says, "You're right, I do feel a lot more relaxed." She sits up and you notice that her cheeks are flushed. As you leave the exam room, you tell her to make an appointment at the desk to see you again soon.

AFTERWARD, tell your man that you don't know where he went to medical school, but that you'd like to congratulate the faculty for its excellence in teaching. Tell him how good he made you feel, and how much fun you have with him. Share a good laugh about the fantasy you've just enjoyed. And remember that the smile on his face is for you, not for his lucky patient.

SEXY SNIPPETS

1. *She's staring at the ceiling in the small exam room as you massage the soft mounds of her breasts, pinching the hard nipples.*

2. *You push your finger deep into her pussy, and caress it inside in a way you know will arouse her.*

3. *You guide your cock into her wet pussy slowly, trying to hide what you're doing behind the draped sheet.*

4. *She starts to move and twist, trying to fight the arousal she's feeling.*

5. *You steady yourself as your orgasm builds, and the come jets out of your cock into her.*

7

THE LAP DANCE

ANY MEN have been to see strippers. Some have had lap dances. Few have had sex with the stripper or the dancer. But after this fantasy, your partner can boast that he has done it all. And in his own living room! This fantasy demands a little more sexual bravado on your part than do some of the others. Brace yourself. You're going to strip in front of your partner. Oh, yes, you are.

This is one of those fantasies that you might have to convince yourself to begin, but once you get going you'll have a great time. As always, your goal is to explore all aspects of your partner's sexuality. Having a woman strip in front of him and then perform a lap dance would undoubtedly turn your partner on. And it will certainly help to get rid of your own inhibitions.

To get the most out of this fantasy, treat yourself to a sexy new short dress and a new matching bra and panty set. Go for sex appeal, not comfort or practicality, and try a style that you wouldn't normally choose. Unless you're already a DD cup, consider buying a padded and/or push-up bra to really get your man's attention. You want stripper boobs for tonight, so go all out!

Recall the importance of your partner seeing your body in a different way. New clothes will help you achieve this goal. Wear high heels and dark red lipstick. Apply body glitter and use new perfume. You can look for a spray-on type of scented body glitter at the drugstore. These are geared toward young girls, but they're great for women of any age. If you really want to impress him, rent or buy a long wig that is a different color than your hair. These are available for very little at any costume shop.

This fantasy is best played out in the living room, but a kitchen chair will work best, since most lounge-type chairs are too cumbersome to work around. Dim the lights and put on some sexy music that will be easy to move your body to. Don't freak out, you're not going to embarrass yourself. You're going to try something new, have fun, and show your partner a good time.

Reassure yourself that you don't need to amaze him with a dazzling dance or strip routine. Just move your body. The moves suggested here are fairly easy to do, but don't hesitate to do what feels right, or what he'd like to see you do. Nobody is judging you, especially not your man—he'll be too busy enjoying himself. Think you're too fat or too old to strip? Think again. Chances are, your partner isn't Hollywood Hunk material either. And who cares anyway? Sex doesn't feel any better for the beautiful people.

Remember at all times that your body is the only near-naked female body in the room—so use it! If you feel silly doing this, use the silliness to your advantage. Laughter and fun are incredibly sexy things, so laugh at yourself and be a good sport. Good sexual sportsmanship is always desirable, and is the right attitude to adopt in order to get the most out of fantasies.

Sometime during the day, send an unexpected sexy message to your partner at work. You can send a suggestive e-mail or leave a throaty message on his voicemail. Cut out a naked picture from a favorite magazine, if that's your style, and discreetly slip it into his pocket or lunch box before he heads off in the morning. Whatever you do, make sure he's thinking sexy thoughts throughout the day so that he'll anticipate coming home to you.

Tell him something like:

When you get home, you're in for a show.

Let his mind wander.

You can either greet your partner at the door wearing your new sexy outfit, or you can secretly change into it later in the evening. In any case, be sure that you have prepared both yourself and your surroundings before you lead him into the living room. When you're ready, have him sit in the chair. You can offer him a drink to enjoy as he watches you. You can also place a roll of dollar bills in his pocket and encourage him to play along by tucking these into your bra and panties when you do something he likes.

Begin to move your body to the music. If you're feeling awkward or embarrassed, just go with it, giggle, and watch as your partner does the same. Set the mood by having fun and not taking what you're doing too seriously.

Once you're ready, you can whisper about what's in store for him.

Tonight I want you to imagine that you're in a seedy bar or a strip club, sitting and watching the girls on the stage move and dance. One of the girls notices you looking at her, and slowly comes closer to you. She's wearing a little dress, and she begins to peel it off right in front of you.

Take some time to remove your dress. You want him to anticipate your every move. Pull the bottom of the dress up slowly while moving your hips sexily.

This girl has decided that she wants to give you a show, up close and personal.

Pull your dress over your head in one motion so your partner gets a visual blast of you wearing only your push-up bra and skimpy panties. Let him savor the sight of your breasts at their absolute best. He will also enjoy the glitter of your body and the scent of your perfume as you move closer to him.

Continue to move your hips and your whole body slowly and seductively all around your man while he sits in the chair. Spend some time in front of him, then slink behind him and rub his shoulders. Press your breasts into his back and wrap your arms around his neck from behind. Reach down and rub your hands all over his chest. Breathe heavily into his ear, and kiss him lightly on the neck.

When you're in front of him again, begin to touch yourself all over your body. This may be difficult for you to do at first, but it is almost guaranteed to arouse your partner. Men love to see women touch themselves. As always, seeing your partner's reaction will make it easier for you, and will arouse you as well.

Lean your head back and sexily drag your fingers down your neck. Push your chest out, take a breast in each hand, and squeeze. Show him that it feels good. If you immerse yourself in the role, it *will* feel good. Pretend you're a sexy, irresistible, and talented lap dancer. You'll turn both of you on. Run your hands all over your stomach and hips and down your thighs, moving and gyrating the whole time. Be bold. Cup your vagina and rock your hips back and forth into your own hand.

This girl's decided to give you a lap dance, but there are very strict rules. She can touch you, but you can't touch her. The manager is very adamant that customers don't touch his girls. You just sit tight.

Accept that your lap dance is not going to be as flawlessly choreographed as a professional's, and remind yourself that it doesn't have to be. Turn your back on your partner, and position yourself as if you're going to simply sit down on his lap. Put your hands on your hips and move them in a circular motion, being sure to thrust your bottom close to his face in a teasing way.

Hook your thumbs into the sides of your panties and pull them down over your buttocks so that your bare bum is close to your man's face. Pull your panties back up. Continue to move your hips in a circle and slowly lower your bum until it touches your partner's lap. Brush it lightly over his lap as best you can.

Turn and face your partner, spreading his legs far apart. Position yourself between his legs and move your body up and down, close to his but not touching. Cup and squeeze your breasts and bring them close to his face. Pull back a bit. Arch your back, stick your chest out, and hook your thumbs under your bra's shoulder straps. Pull the straps down and let your breasts burst out of the bra. Don't take your bra off completely, just leave it hanging fastened around your ribs. Run your hands over your partner's chest and thighs.

If your agility and the chair's constitution will permit it, straddle your man on the chair and arch your back so that your breasts are close to his face. Rock back and forth on his lap. If you aren't able to sit on him, just remain between his legs and brush your body up and down against his.

Continue with the story.

You can feel yourself getting hard, and you're dreading that she's going to get you all worked up, and then you'll have to leave feeling so unsatisfied. You're almost wishing you were already home so you could think about this and jerk off. You know you will as soon as you get in the door.

Lean in close and whisper into your partner's ear.

You can tell this girl is actually getting turned on. She's thinking that she'd like to give you a little something extra tonight. A dance won't cut it. She needs the real thing tonight, not just teasing. Imagine that the place is empty, all the other customers have left. This girl knows that nobody, including her boss, will find out if she gives a customer a little more. Anyway, lots of the girls do it, and sometimes the boss even suggests they should. It's good for business. Lots of repeat customers.

Climb off your partner and kneel between his spread legs. Undo his pants and pull them and his underwear down. Stand, turn your back on him, and pull your panties down. Brush your bare bum over his lap. Take your panties right off. Turn around again to face him.

It would be a completely unexpected and delicious delicacy for your man if you have removed your pubic hair. What are you using it for anyway? If you don't want to remove it completely, leave just a little tuft. The more you can use your body to thrill your partner, the more thrill you will receive in return.

Move your body against your man's in any and all ways that make him hard. Tease him, and make him long for the release only you can give him. When it's time to build your mutual orgasms, decide how you want to proceed.

If you are able to sit on your partner's lap on the chair, climb on top of him and lower yourself onto his stiff penis.

You can't believe it, but this girl is sitting on top of you, fucking you. Every now and then she leans close and hotly whispers into your ear, "Don't touch me . . . you're not allowed to use your hands." She tells you how she felt your hardness when she was rubbing against you, and that turned her on so much . . . she has to use you to satisfy herself.

Move up and down, rocking your body and pressing your breasts into your partner's face. Remember to moan and arch your back. Give him a real show.

She wants to get off on you. She just wants to use you, and she wants to come on you.

Make yourself come, and make the most of it. If you aren't ready, fake it. Forget what you've heard about faking it— sometimes it's a terrifically effective thing. It takes the "pressure" off, and allows both of you to relax and reach orgasm. Faking it is just one more sexual technique at your disposal. And it doesn't mean you won't reach real orgasm yourself. You can let him think he's given you multiple orgasms once you reach the real thing.

This girl came so hard on your cock. Now she wants you to

come. She wants to feel that hot liquid jet inside her and fill her up. She wants to feel your wonderful wet warmth run over her clit and down her thighs afterward.

Talk like a stripper. Talking dirty is another weapon in your sexual arsenal, and if not used too frequently, it is a powerful one. Continue until your partner comes.

If you prefer, you can make your partner every bit as happy by performing oral sex. Kneel between his spread legs and begin to lick and kiss his thighs. Increase your urgency as you get closer and closer to his penis. Make him think that you can't wait to put it in your mouth. And remind him often that he's not allowed to use his hands.

This girl's on a mission. She wants to make you come as hard as you can inside her mouth. She wants to feel your come shoot into her mouth and slide down her throat, and she needs to swallow every drop to satisfy her craving. She felt your hardness when she was rubbing against you, and she couldn't stop thinking about how good it would feel in her mouth. She couldn't wait to see it.

Without using your hands, take your partner's penis in your mouth and bob your head back and forth on it. Lick it, then suck both softly and strongly to make it as hard as possible. Lick and suck his perineum, testicles, and frenulum, going from one to the other in sequence, slowly and then quickly. You will have to nuzzle your face right in there, since your hands should be busy grabbing and rubbing his legs and thighs. Moan, moan, moan.

When your partner is ready to build the momentum he needs to orgasm, adopt a more steady rhythm and pace to accommodate him. Don't stop until he comes. Let him ejaculate

into your mouth and don't let up on his penis until he is finished. Keep sucking or stroking his penis until he tells you to
stop, since the sensation lasts beyond the orgasm.

*You feel your orgasm build as your cock disappears again
and again into the girl's hot mouth. Her hands are desperately
clutching your thighs as she brings you closer to release. The
feeling finally peaks and a strong orgasm runs through your
body. The girl keeps sucking until the feeling subsides and
you're completely content.*

*You sit back in the chair in happy exhaustion. The girl gath-
ers her clothes off the floor and hastily dresses. She collects the
money lying on the floor, but slips it into your pocket with a
smile. "Your shows will always be free, mister."*

AFTERWARD, share a laugh with your partner about your
performance and thank him for making you feel comfortable
enough to get over your stage fright. Tell him you enjoyed
making him feel good, and that he made you come really
hard. Tell him that if you had to choose any lap anywhere in
the world to squirm around on, it would be his. Pat yourself
on the back for your bravery, for pleasing your partner in this
new way, and for bringing this erotic and fun experience into
your sex life. There's so much more to sexual fantasies than
bringing your partner to orgasm. Having fun together is a
huge part of it, and it's also the essence of a long and happy
relationship. And remember that the smile on your man's
face as he watches you gather your clothes off the floor is for
you, not for the saucy stripper.

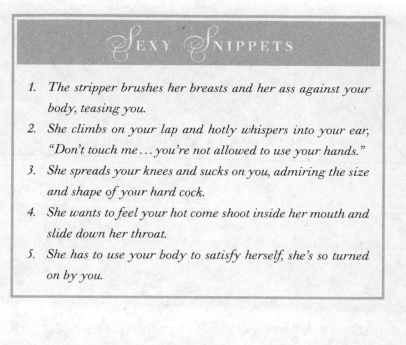

Sexy Snippets

1. The stripper brushes her breasts and her ass against your body, teasing you.
2. She climbs on your lap and hotly whispers into your ear, "Don't touch me...you're not allowed to use your hands."
3. She spreads your knees and sucks on you, admiring the size and shape of your hard cock.
4. She wants to feel your hot come shoot inside her mouth and slide down her throat.
5. She has to use your body to satisfy herself, she's so turned on by you.

8

THE PAJAMA PARTY

H, THE PAJAMA PARTY. It is the essence of girl-ish fun and innocence. But not in this book, it isn't. In this fantasy, your partner finds himself at the mercy of a lustful mob of coeds. He is the innocent, unsuspecting workman held hostage at a college sorority pajama party. You can imagine that these girls are clinging to academic life at the bottom of the curve. They see your virtuous guy, and they want him to be their next sexual casualty. The poor dear. This is a classic example of being in the wrong place at the right time.

If you choose to simply whisper the details of this fantasy into your partner's ear, that's fine. However, if you choose to role-play and act parts of it out, this fantasy will let your part-ner experience sex in a very different way.

In this love scene, he will be blindfolded and gagged. His inability to see in advance what his body is going to feel, or to watch it happening, will dramatically increase both the level of his arousal and the enjoyment of this fantasy. The strangely invasive sensation of the gag in his mouth, combined with the feeling of helplessness it fosters, will turn him on and help bring the fantasy to life in his mind. Your partner will love the unfamiliar way sex feels when his senses are restricted in this way. And you will love the sense of sexual control as you do to him whatever you wish.

Instead of coming to bed in your usual scrubs, purchase new pajamas. Buy something you wouldn't ordinarily choose so that your man will see you in a different way. Something girlish is best for this fantasy, such as a sheer teddy with frills, or a cute T-shirt-and-shorts outfit. If you have an oversized college sweatshirt or T-shirt, go bare-legged in that.

You want to set a scene of girlish fun and games in this sexy sorority house so that your partner can clearly visualize it. In addition to the changes to your bedclothes, try throwing a few fluffy oversized pillows on your bed to romp around on. You'll need a chair in your bedroom, since he will be tied to that before moving to the bed. Have a few scarves or ties handy, for binding him to the bedposts. If you don't have bedposts, you can tie his wrists together and put his arms over his head for essentially the same effect. You'll also need something to use as a blindfold and a gag.

If you want, you can stage this fantasy in your living room instead of your bedroom. You can tie your partner to a chair and then restrain him on the floor by tying him to the legs of the couch and coffee table. Go ahead and amend the script to your own convenience.

If you're going to have dinner before engaging in this fantasy, serve true college cuisine. Make macaroni and cheese, or

order in a pizza. You can eat in your pajamas to let your partner enjoy the sight of you in them, or you can change into
them before the fantasy begins. The food and the pajamas
will give you an opening into this fantasy; in fact, your partner will likely clue in quickly to what you're doing, especially
if you've played with fantasies in the past.

You can say something like:

*I was talking to So-and-so at work today, and she was telling
me about her daughter who's in college. She was saying how
much more worldly college students are today than we were at
their age. She said her daughter has a new boyfriend every time
she turns around, and that she knows she's sexually active with
all of them. Do you think it's the freedom of college life that
makes some girls so promiscuous, or is it just a generational
thing? Or maybe some girls have always been like that.*

*Anyway, it got me thinking and my mind started wander-
ing. I started to think about what goes on behind closed doors in
some of those college sororities and dormitories. All those girls
free for the first time to explore and experiment with sex without their parents around. I'm sure some of them take it to ex-
tremes and get pretty carried away. I can imagine what they
talk about when they all get together! Girls talk a lot more and
a lot more graphically about sex than men think they do, you
know.*

Your partner may be interested to learn just how openly
and how often girls talk about sex when they get together.
This conversation may be enough to turn him on, or at least
get him thinking in a sexual way.

It's now time to have him visualize the scene. Twirl your
hair, or his, in your fingers while you speak. Tickle his scalp
or body. Suck or play with his fingers and toes. Flirt, and do

anything that he finds fun or amusing—it will set the mood for this mischievous story.

Can you imagine a group of college girls, all hanging out late at night at their sorority house? They're having a pajama party. Everywhere you look there are girls running around in skimpy little pajamas ... short see-through teddies, bikini panties and bras, and tight cotton T-shirts. Some are just wearing baggy sweatshirts or T-shirts with smooth, bare legs.

They're all giggling and telling stories about sex. They're talking about sexual encounters they've had. They're talking about things they did to boys, things boys did to them, and things they'd still like to try. There are no boys there, but some of the girls are saying how much they wish there were. All that talk about sex is turning them on.

Now that you've set the stage, have your partner visualize himself on it.

Imagine you're a workman and you've been called out late at night to fix a furnace, and you end up at the wrong house. You knock on the door of this sorority and a girl answers. She's wearing a thin, see-through blue teddy. It barely covers her crotch, and her nipples are clearly visible underneath. Her hair is up in a ponytail, and as soon as she opens the door you know you've come to the wrong place.

You've mistakenly come to a sorority, but on the outside it just looked like a regular house. You're embarrassed, and you glance behind her to see girls everywhere. They're barely clothed and they're running around giggling. The girl at the door gives you a wide smile. You apologize sheepishly and tell her you have the wrong address.

You turn to go but suddenly you feel hands grabbing at you and pulling you inside the house. The door slams behind you.

You're stunned that these girls have physically forced you inside this house. You're a strong man, but you can't fight off the ten or twelve girls that start dragging you across the floor. At first you're hesitant to be physical with them in case you hurt them, but soon you're struggling as hard as you can to get away.

Snuggle in close to your partner and begin to move your hands all over his body. Use more pressure than you usually would, to emphasize the physicality of what is happening to him in the fantasy.

You can barely comprehend what is happening to you. You don't know if this is a joke or some sort of college prank. There's music pounding in the background and you don't know if you should be scared or what. The girls roughly sit you on a chair. Several of them hold you down while some others scurry around looking for something to tie you up with. Before you know it, you're bound tightly to the chair and you can't move.

Persuade your partner to let you similarly tie him to a chair. By this time he should know what you have planned for him this evening, and will likely be a willing victim. Bind his wrists and his ankles to the chair as tightly as he is comfortable with.

You shake your head frantically as a couple of the girls struggle to put a blindfold over your eyes. Before you know it the room has gone pitch black. You can't see a thing. You're tied very tightly to the chair, and the physical restraint is quickly making you angry. You don't care anymore if this is a prank. You shout for somebody to untie you and to take the blindfold off your eyes.

In response, you feel a cloth around your mouth. You realize they're gagging you. They tie the gag behind your head. A feeling of helplessness creeps over you as you picture yourself in the middle of this room at the mercy of these girls, bound to a chair, blindfolded and gagged.

Begin to blindfold and gag your man while you are relating this part of the fantasy. Be gentle with him and tell him you're not going to do anything he doesn't like. You're just going to have a little fun. Tell him that you're going to tie him loosely enough for him to easily break free and remove the blindfold and gag. The very process of being restrained in this way will probably turn him on, and chances are he will be far more aroused and curious than worried or hesitant.

At this point he'll be restrained on the chair and won't be able to see what you're doing, or to respond verbally. This is exactly where and how you want him. You can now do things he won't be able to see coming. The anticipation of where and when your touch will come will be thrilling to both of you!

You can hear the girls laughing. You can hear the pounding music, and you can hear your own muffled grunts of protest. You're not really scared, you just want to free yourself. You know they're not going to hurt you, but you're surprised at their audacity. You stop struggling and wait for them to come to their senses and release you.

You're expecting to feel the restraints loosen or the blindfold lift at any moment, but instead you feel something brushing against your lips. You can't identify what it is at first. Then you feel more things brushing against your lips and moving lightly all over your face.

Take off your top and drag your nipples all over your partner's face and mouth, doing whatever feels good. Place one of them in his mouth as best you can around the gag.

Don't tell him what is happening, just let him figure it out.

The same strategy goes for everything you will do to your man in this fantasy. Let his senses absorb the physical sensations you provide, but leave him to figure out exactly what you are doing. Bathe him in the unexpected and unseen sexual sensations washing over his body. If he knows what is coming, his body will be prepared for it and the sexual impact will be diminished. You want him to imagine he is at the mercy of these girls, and that he doesn't know what they are going to do to him. They're not telling, so neither should you.

Unzip your partner's jeans and gently free his penis. Touch it lightly and teasingly, and then begin to perform oral sex on him.

Imagine yourself tied to this chair, completely helpless, and these girls are doing whatever they want to you. You're at their mercy and the more they touch you, the more aroused you become. You can feel so much stimulation on your cock, but you can't see exactly what they're doing.

You don't want to get hard, but you can feel your body betraying you. Whatever they're doing feels so good that you are responding involuntarily, even though you try to stop it. You don't want to get turned on and you definitely don't want them to see you get hard. Your body has no right to betray you like this, but their eager mouths on your cock send shivers up your spine.

Out of the many voices you can hear around you, one is speaking to you. A girl tells you that she and her sorority sisters are going to have a little contest, and you're going to be the judge. You're going to pick the winner.

You must now pretend that you are three different girls competing to perform the best oral sex on your partner. Use three very different oral techniques. For example, you can deep-throat softly as far as you can with the first; squeeze tightly with the second, using your tongue to lick and flick around the testicles, perineum, shaft, frenulum, and head; and then suck hard with the third.

Be sure to make each technique different enough to be recognizably distinct. Pause between each to let your partner imagine the girls are changing places. Ask your partner which girl has the best technique.

The girls decide to move you onto the floor. They want to tie you to the legs of the coffee table and the couch so that you'll be spread wide open for them to look at and touch. They want you completely naked. They want to force you into the most vulnerable position they can, and do whatever they want to you.

Untie your partner's wrists and ankles and, while he is still blindfolded and gagged, undress him roughly.

Imagine all these girls are roughly tearing your clothes off of you. You feel totally exposed.

Have your partner lie flat on the bed or the floor, wherever you are best able to tie him spread-eagle. Again, tell him that you are going to tie him loosely enough for him to break free at any time.

Once your partner is lying naked, flat on his back with his arms and legs spread open and restrained, ensure that he has a good visual sense of his new circumstances by re-describing his situation. Don't be afraid to do this often in order to refresh his memory and appeal to his mind's eye. Take a long look at him in this state. It will be arousing to see him so vulnerable and so turned on!

Imagine yourself blindfolded and gagged, lying flat on your back on the floor of this strange house. Your clothes have been torn off against your will, and you're helpless and exposed.

You're tied tightly by your wrists and ankles. Your arms are wide open. Your legs are spread wide and your cock is out in the open for all those girls to see. You can feel the weight of their stares on it, and against your will it gets harder and harder. You can feel it sticking up into the air and you know they're looking at it.

Take off any remaining clothes you have on and straddle your partner. Without telling him in advance, lower yourself onto his penis. Start slowly, then bounce up and down enthusiastically. Since you want him to picture girl after girl having sex with him, repeatedly climb off and back on him. Each time you climb on him and lower yourself onto his penis, make a different sound and move your body in a different rhythm and intensity to create the impression of multiple girls.

You can't see, you can't speak, and you can't move a muscle. One by one the girls take turns fucking you. Imagine your body being used by all these girls to get themselves off. You never know who is on you or what she looks like. Once in a while you feel a shudder above you and you know you're making them come.

Close your eyes and really picture this scene playing out. Let yourself come whenever you like, and keep climbing off and on until your partner is ready to have an orgasm too.

When you can tell he is close to coming, say something like:

These girls are rough, as though they're using you. But your cock loves them anyway. It's throbbing and pulsing with such intensity that it hurts. As each tight, wet pussy slams down on it, you feel your orgasm building. Finally, you feel the release. You feel the come shoot out with a force you've never felt before.

Your body jerks and spasms as the come jets out, again and again. The girl on top of you feels it too, and she grinds her pussy down on top of you as hard as she can.

Let your partner come inside.

A warm sense of pleasure spreads through your body as your orgasm subsides. The girl climbs off of you and releases you from your bonds. The coeds all offer you mischievous smiles and you grin back at them. After they give you a slice of pizza to replenish yourself, they send you on your way, telling you that you're always welcome at their sorority. You assure them you'll be back soon to check their furnace, free of charge.

AFTERWARD, tell your man that if you had your choice of any workman to tie to the coffee table, it would be him. Tell him how hard he got and how good he felt inside you. Tell him you couldn't believe how powerfully he came and that you love it when you feel that warmth inside you. If you didn't eat beforehand, or if you're ready to be replenished, order a pizza. Your partner may have to refuel after being subjected to the whims of so many college girls. Massage his hands and feet to help him wind down from fantasy mode and to pleasantly send him off to sleep. And remember that the smile on his face (when you remove the gag!) is for you, not for the sexy sorority sisters.

*S*EXY *S*NIPPETS

1. *You're surrounded by these girls, they're dressed in T-shirts and see-through teddies.*
2. *You can feel their hard nipples dragging along your bare skin.*
3. *You're tied up, and you can't see or speak. The girls are taking turns, competing to suck you the best.*
4. *You're on your back and the girls are lowering themselves onto you . . . you can feel them coming on your cock, one after the other.*
5. *You feel your orgasm building as each tight, warm, wet pussy slams down on your cock.*

9

THE VERY PERSONAL DEMO

HAVE YOU EVER gone into a sex shop? Love bou-tique? Adult novelty store? Marital aid center? A rose by any other name would carry the same array of toys, gadgets, and magic potions. If you have visited such a place, no doubt you wandered down the aisles filled with curiosity and sometimes awe. You also probably wondered in amaze-ment exactly how some mystery items were to be used by an anatomically correct human in safety and comfort.

If you are lucky, the clerk might discreetly educate you while you dodge direct eye contact. If not, you can buy it caveat emptor and hope for the best. But what would happen if your partner were to receive a personal demonstration from the attractive but somewhat too-helpful lady clerk? In this fantasy, he'll find out. Do you think the combined effect of stealing away in the middle of the day to visit a sex shop, the strange sex paraphernalia all around him, and the frank sexual talk and demonstrations of a stranger could excite him? Let's hope so.

This fantasy will arouse your man whether you choose to whisper the details and dialogue into his ear, or whether you choose to act part of it out. If you choose the latter, this fantasy requires some fortitude on your part—specifically, a visit to a sex shop. If you have visited one in the past, you already know it's no big deal. If you haven't, relax. The clerks have seen and heard it all. They've seen fat and slim, married and unmarried, gay and straight, the informed and the wildly ignorant, the bold and the meek, the lone and the accompanied, and they don't bat an eyelid. There is absolutely nothing to be embarrassed about. Keep in mind that the reason there are so many sex shops is because so many people visit them. The law of supply and demand ensures that you are not alone.

Your shopping list for this fantasy may include any or all of the following: a dildo, a vibrator, special condoms, wrist and ankle restraints, nipple clamps, some type of slapper, a cock ring, ben wa balls, a blindfold, a feather, a book on sexual positions, and edible flavored body lotion. There is a seemingly unlimited arsenal of these items, so the size or style of each is up to you. If you see anything else that catches your eye, go ahead and buy it.

The great thing about this fantasy is its versatility. You can easily tailor this fantasy around your purchases simply by substituting them in your personalized version. For the purposes of this fantasy, only a few of the more usual and comparatively tame items listed above will be featured. In all likelihood your plot won't involve all of them since they can be quite costly, but bear in mind that quality is more important than quantity. Your partner will enjoy this fantasy just as much with three items as he will with thirty. It's your imaginations that you're appealing to, and it will only take a few novelty items to fire those up.

With your new toys safely hidden underneath your pillow, crawl into bed with your partner.

Ease into the fantasy by stirring your partner's curiosity. Say something like:

I made a stop today at a very special place... I wanted to get you something you could enjoy. I walked up and down the aisles looking for something, but I was too embarrassed to buy half the stuff and I wasn't sure how to use the other half!

After he tunes in to the fact that you visited a sex shop, you can add a little friendly fabrication. Nuzzle into his neck, and say:

It was in the middle of the day, so it was pretty empty in there. I got in and out pretty fast, but there was one other guy in there that seemed to be stalling. I think he was waiting for me to leave before he could bring himself to look at the stuff. Come to think of it, the lady clerk rang me through rather quickly. Maybe I interrupted something. It's easy to get a little turned on looking at some of that stuff, maybe her work was getting to her. Maybe she was trying out some new inventory on him or giving him a personal demonstration of how some of those things work. The guy probably couldn't believe his luck. You know?

Up until now you've been telling your story casually, but now you should have your partner actively picture the scene.

Imagine you went into a sex shop in the middle of the afternoon. There's nobody else in there except the clerk. She's very pretty and you're a little uncomfortable when you first walk

*in. You remind yourself that she's seen it all and you begin
looking around. There are pictures everywhere of naked
women in all sorts of poses. Some of the pictures show women
and men together.*

*Everywhere you look you see images of naked bodies, sex,
and blow jobs. You can't help but get a little aroused, but it's
such a public place that you manage to keep yourself in check.
You're standing in front of a wall that's covered with dildos and
images of women using them on each other, men using them
on women, and even women using them on men. You're an experienced guy, but you're a little embarrassed by the graphic
pictures.*

Begin to caress your man's body as you describe the interior of the sex shop. You should also be actively visualizing
the shop and its products. You want to arouse yourself and
immerse yourself in your role as the very friendly clerk.
Imagine you've been surrounded by sexual images and toys
all day, and now this handsome, virile man has wandered in.

*Imagine that the clerk comes up to you from behind and asks
you if you need any help. She's very friendly and she makes
you feel comfortable right away, despite the awkwardness of
your surroundings. You smile and tell her that you're looking
for something fun for you and your girlfriend…for some reason you want her to know that you have a girlfriend. Maybe she
won't think you're such a pervert if she knows you're shopping
for two. She tells you there are lots of fun things for couples, and
asks you if you've used any toys before. You tell her you haven't.
She smiles and tells you that you're in for a good time.*

Grin, and touch your partner's lips, or give him a light kiss
as you describe the clerk's scampish smile.

The clerk tells you to follow her, and she walks briskly around the store, up and down the aisles, snatching things off the shelves as she goes along. She takes you and the merchandise to the back of the store where a dark blue curtain is pulled across a doorway. You get the sense it's a changing room or something. She pulls the curtain back and both of you step into a small windowless room. She pulls the curtain closed behind you.

You're wondering what's going on, and she tells you that since you haven't used any toys before, she's going to show you how they work. She says you're lucky because the store is so quiet she's able to take the time to give you a personal demonstration. She doesn't want you to fumble around when you get home. She wants you to be able to turn your girlfriend on with these things, so you'll need a little practice.

Refresh your partner's visualization of where he is and what is happening. Touch his shoulders and brush your fingers on his cheek. Start to wake up his skin and his body.

Imagine yourself in this secret room tucked into the back of a sex shop, illuminated with fluorescent lights. The clerk piles all the merchandise on a chair in the corner of the room and sifts through it. She's going to show you how these sex toys work. She is very matter-of-fact, and doesn't seem to think that this is at all strange. It's just good customer service—she's done it a thousand times.

The first thing she picks up to show you is a vibrator. It's a basic straight one, shiny red and smooth. She turns the dial at the bottom and you hear a bzzzz. She begins to run it over her hands, and then takes your hands to show you how it feels.

You should now pull out your hidden vibrator and begin to

rub it over your partner's hands. This will surprise him, and it won't break fantasy mode to share a laugh!

She says, "Doesn't that feel goods?... This is how you should use it on your girlfriend." She takes the vibrator and begins to run it along her thighs. Several times she comes close to running it between her legs, but stops and says, "Tease her a little... make her really want to feel it down there."

Kneel on the bed beside him and rub yourself with the vibrator in a like manner. Do what feels good, and let him see you becoming aroused. If you or your partner is turned on by it, let him watch as you insert the vibrator into your vagina.

Finally, she pushes it between her long legs. She spreads them open more, and you watch as she rubs and pokes herself with the vibrating rod. "This feels so nice... your girlfriend will love it... are you watching how I'm doing it? It will feel good for you to use it, too." She pulls it away from herself and begins to lightly rub your groin with it, through your jeans.

Run the vibrator lightly over your man's penis and testicles, through his underwear.

You feel an instant surge of arousal as this strange woman strokes you with the vibrator. She stops just as quickly, and turns back to the pile of goods on the chair.

"Here's something she'll really enjoy, although they take some getting used to... they're nipple clamps. I'll show you how they go on." As if it's nothing unusual, the clerk pulls her shirt off over her head and exposes her bare breasts. You feel a sudden throb in your cock. The whole idea of where you are and what you're doing is beginning to sink in.

Still kneeling, pull out the hidden nipple clamps and pull off your top. It may be a surprise treat if you have applied some body glitter (perhaps that which you used in the lap dance fantasy) to your breasts. Continue to do what you're describing the clerk as doing.

She says, "it's best if you can get the nipples a bit hard first," and she tweaks one of her nipples with her fingers. "Mmmm, that feels good." You're getting so turned on that you're holding your breath, waiting anxiously to see what she'll do next.

You watch as the clerk bites her lower lip and gently places a clamp on her nipple. She draws her breath at a twinge of pain, but then leans her head back with a satisfied, sensual smile. She tells you to look closely at her nipple to see how the clamp is properly applied. She places the second clamp on her other nipple. She puts both her hands on the back of her head and shakes her breasts around. "Make sure she moves like this to get the full effect... god, these things are great if your nipples are sensitive like mine are."

Remember that many men love to watch women touch and stimulate themselves. Continue to act out the fantasy by using your new toys on yourself and on your partner.

The clerk takes off the nipple clamps and picks up a cock ring. "This kind of cock ring goes around both your penis and your testicles... you can't return it, so we'd better make sure that this one fits you." She casually reaches out and undoes your jeans, letting them fall to the floor. Before you can even register what she's doing, your underwear is also lying on the floor.

Remove your partner's underwear. Take a moment to admire how attractive his penis and testicles are, and make sure he can see your admiration.

"Wow, your girlfriend is a lucky lady." The air hits your cock and you watch it harden before your eyes. "Oh good, it's easier if you're already a bit hard." She wraps the cock ring around your privates and right away you feel the blood pound-

ing in your rapidly swelling dick. "This will keep you hard a long time so your girlfriend can really get her money's worth out of you!"

The clerk turns back to the chair and picks up some little metal balls. She tells you that they're called ben wa balls, and that your girlfriend can put them in her vagina and leave them there as long as she wants. You open your eyes wide as she pulls down her pants and panties and steps out of them to reveal her pussy. It's shaved into a thin racing stripe. "She can put one leg up on a chair to insert them, or she can lie down and do it . . . or you can do it for her . . . here, I'll lie down and you put them into practice."

Lie down and let your partner insert the ben wa balls into your vagina. Be vocal and let him know how incredibly good they feel. Remember that he will be more turned on knowing that *you* are turned on. If you aren't comfortable using this or any type of sex toy, no matter. Either substitute something you are okay with, or just describe rather than perform that part of the fantasy. There are always options.

The clerk lies on her back and spreads her knees apart. You kneel between her legs and stare at her pussy while you push the balls past the soft lips and into it. She squirms around a bit, and then asks you to take them out. You're rock-hard now. You remove the balls, and you know they felt good because they're slick with her juice. Her pussy looks irresistibly inviting. You're torn between making a move on her right there, or getting out as fast as you can so you can jerk off in the car. You know you have to do something soon . . . your body is straining and your balls are throbbing with a dull, pleasurable ache.

The clerk gets up and picks up a dildo and some flavored

body gel. "The great thing about a dildo is that you can be fucking your girlfriend while she gives you a blow job at the same time... I can show you how my boyfriend and I do it, if you want." You're afraid your voice will crack if you answer, so you just nod. She hands you the dildo. "Okay, you lie on the floor and I'll pretend I'm her. It's like we're going to sixty-nine... I get on top of you so that I can suck your dick and you can easily insert the dildo in me. You should get some of this flavored body gel so she can put it on you. There are lots of flavors and they're really good."

You and your partner should now get into a sixty-nine position, you spreading gel on his penis and him holding the dildo. You can use the vibrator instead of the dildo, if you prefer.

You lie on the floor and feel a rush of pleasure as the clerk rubs some of the gel onto you. You stare at the ceiling and are struck by an intense wave of arousal as you notice that a mirror has been placed up there. You can clearly see the woman on top of you, spreading the gel on your stiff shaft. You can see yourself under her, holding the dildo and ready to push it in her.

She tells you to push the dildo inside her, and when you do she lets out a loud moan and leans back into it. She moves herself back and forth on the dildo, then tells you to begin moving it in and out of her. As you begin to do this, she wraps her hot mouth tightly around your cock and begins to suck it. You're so close to coming that you try to push her off of you, but she holds on tight and keeps sucking. She wants you to experience an orgasm with the cock ring on.

Your partner might half-heartedly push you away, but hold

on and keep sucking. This in itself should make him come, and if you want him to ejaculate in your mouth, continue sucking on him until he does.

Give him a good image of what he is seeing in the fantasy mirror overhead.

You stare into the mirror on the ceiling as you fuck this woman in her mouth with your cock, and in her pussy with the dildo. It's an incredible sight, this naked woman on top of you... the harder you push the dildo in, the harder she sucks. You stare into the mirror and watch the back of her head bob up and down as she swallows your entire length again and again in her mouth.

Remember that the great thing about you leading your man through these fantasies is that very often you get to decide how you want him, and you, to come. Do what you crave, since if you're having a good time, he'll have a good time. Accordingly, if you want your partner inside you, and don't want him to ejaculate in your mouth, stop sucking and say something like:

The clerk climbs off of you and kneels on the floor. She says, "I want you to experience what it's like to get off with the cock ring on before you try it on your girlfriend... why don't you go ahead and try it on me? I hope you don't mind, but I only let customers do me from behind, it's less personal that way."

Kneel on the bed and let your partner penetrate you from behind. Remind him once again of the ceiling mirror so he can visualize himself in it. It shouldn't take long for either of you to come at this point.

You lean your head back on your shoulders and stare up into the mirror on the ceiling... the woman is on her hands and knees and you're pounding into her from behind. You're grip-

ping her hips tightly and pulling her body back hard onto your swollen dick. Her breasts shake and her whole body jolts forward each time you pound into her. You see your cock disappear into her pussy, and you hear the slapping sound of your body against her ass every time you push into her. You can feel your orgasm building. You're hitting her so fast that you can't even count your thrusts.

Push yourself back against your man's body to meet each of his thrusts. Let yourself moan when he comes, and grind your bum against his body so he knows you like the sensation of him coming inside you. Be sure to remove the cock ring soon after he ejaculates.

You come together, and as you do, the store door chimes to indicate that someone has entered the shop. The clerk giggles and says, "Perfect timing." She quickly makes herself presentable, then darts out of the little room to help her next lucky customer. You lie against the wall in exhaustion, looking at the toys around you. You can't wait to get home and try them out on your girlfriend—now that you know how they work.

AFTERWARD, tell your partner how much fun you had and that you hope he enjoyed this fantasy. Clean your toys well and tuck them away so they don't accidentally turn up at your son's elementary school for show-and-tell. It may amuse him if you have purchased a box you can use as your own "toy box." You can personalize it with your names or a design that is meaningful to you as a couple, and pile all your new toys into it after sex.

Whenever possible, take advantage of the time after sex to do something fun or special as a couple. This doesn't have to be anything elaborate; racing out of bed to raid the fridge or catch the last fifteen minutes of a television show will do. Finally, remember that the smile on your man's face is for you, not for the salesgirl at the local sex shop.

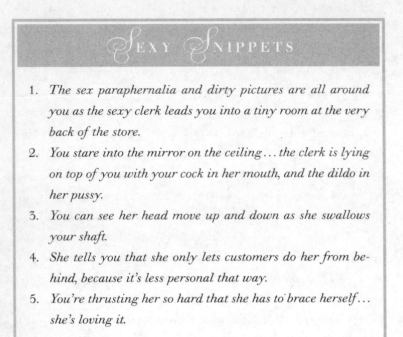

SEXY SNIPPETS

1. *The sex paraphernalia and dirty pictures are all around you as the sexy clerk leads you into a tiny room at the very back of the store.*

2. *You stare into the mirror on the ceiling...the clerk is lying on top of you with your cock in her mouth, and the dildo in her pussy.*

3. *You can see her head move up and down as she swallows your shaft.*

4. *She tells you that she only lets customers do her from behind, because it's less personal that way.*

5. *You're thrusting her so hard that she has to brace herself... she's loving it.*

10

THE BIRTHDAY PRESENT

*C*LEOPATRA. Was she beautiful? No. Was she irresistible to men? Yes.

The more colorful pages of the history books tell us that Cleopatra realized early on how advantageous her woman's body could be to her political standing. Being above all else a practical girl, Cleopatra hired the finest professionals—namely, Egypt's most skilled prostitutes—to tutor her in the art of sexual seduction. And her ingenuity paid off. As a result of her efforts, she became the wife of Caesar and the Queen of Egypt.

Although we may not have the expertise of highly skilled courtesans at our disposal, we do have the power of sexual fantasy. In this fantasy, you will present your partner with a skillful prostitute for his birthday, and the three of you will have your own private party —with you in charge, of course.

The prostitute will only do to him what you instruct and permit her to do. He'll love this one!

When you're lying in bed next to your partner, tell him about the strategic sexual maneuvers of Cleopatra. He will undoubtedly be amused, and this will start a good conversation.

When the time is right, you can playfully say something like:

I wonder if prostitutes really know anything that the rest of us don't. They've seen more, done it more, but do you think it's anything really different? What if, say for your birthday, I gave you a prostitute? Say we've just finished supper one evening, and the doorbell rings. You answer it, and there's a gorgeous, voluptuous blonde woman standing there. She's wearing a skin-tight red leather skirt and high heels. While you're staring at her in the doorway, I come over and invite her in.

If *you* happen to be a "gorgeous, voluptuous blonde woman," make the prostitute a petite brunette. If you're a petite brunette, make her a redhead. You get the picture.

I turn to you and tell you that this beautiful woman is your birthday present. We've been together a long time and I just want to give you a little treat on your birthday. No strings attached, no jealousy, just a really good time for you. The only condition is that I get to tell her exactly what she can and can't do to you.

As always, make sure your partner knows it's okay for him to think about this. If he seems unsure or hesitant, smile and tell him it's okay. He won't want to hurt your feelings, so let him know that he won't.

Set the scene and assist your man's visualization of it.

Imagine that I lead you and the prostitute into our bedroom.

I tell you to stand by the bed, and I tell her to take her clothes off. She obeys immediately. She pulls her tight shirt over her head and exposes her large, bare breasts. She wriggles out of her tight red skirt and pulls off her little red panties. You're just staring at this unfamiliar woman naked in our bedroom, gawking at her huge breasts and small patch of blonde pubic hair. You can't believe this is happening in your own house.

Whisper this into your partner's ear while you gently caress his body at the same time. Every now and then, place soft kisses on his lips and neck, and flick your tongue in his ear. Cuddle into him close so he'll know you're enthusiastic about leading him through this fantasy.

Then I tell the prostitute to undress you.

When you're ready, undress your partner while you continue to tell the story. Be frisky, and let him know you're having fun.

Say something like:

She unbuttons your shirt and takes it off while you stand unmoving and I watch. She reaches down and undoes your pants. She pushes them and your underwear to the floor. She looks at me for further instructions, and I tell her to come over and undress me. You're left standing beside the bed and watching as the naked prostitute takes my clothes off. I walk over and make you lie down on the bed. It's obvious to all of us that you're already enjoying your birthday present.

Hold the sheets over your body while you wriggle and squirm out of your pajamas and panties. Lift the sheets and let your partner peek at your naked body under the covers. Then continue.

Again the prostitute waits for me to tell her what to do. It's clear that I'm in charge of what's going on. I tell her to get on the bed and kneel between your spread legs. She does. I tell her to lean over and gently drag her nipples all over your chest and face. I tell her to put one of her nipples in your mouth, and then I tell you to suck it. You do, and I can tell you're getting really turned on by the unfamiliar taste of another woman's nipple in your mouth. She sits back up and I climb onto the bed beside you. I tell her to suck my nipples so you can watch, and she does. Imagine lying on the bed watching another woman sucking my nipples. You know I'm a bit shy about it, but that I'm doing it because it'll turn you on.

Drag your nipples across your man's chest and face, and place one in his mouth. Enjoy the sensations and the fantasy. You can imagine either that you're watching the prostitute with your partner, or that you're the prostitute invited into this couple's bed.

I tell you to get up on your knees and straddle the prostitute's body so that you're just above her face. When she's lying underneath you, I gently take your penis and direct it down toward her mouth. I tell her to suck it, and she seems to swallow the whole shaft despite its enormity. She's definitely a professional. She starts sucking you from underneath while you kiss me and rub my breasts. The sensations are overwhelming and you can feel your rock-hard cock throbbing so much it almost hurts. She does it differently than I do, and it feels unexpected and strange.

Have your partner straddle your body while you lie on the bed and perform oral sex on him from underneath. Because you are pretending to be someone else, add some variations to the way you usually do this; use different strokes, apply more or less pressure, deep-throat, use your tongue, vary your speed, and make unfamiliar sounds of excitement.

I tell her to stop, and I get you to lie down again.

Have your partner change his position by lying down on the bed. He can now enjoy oral sex in this position while imagining he is receiving it from two women.

I spread your legs wide and then both the prostitute and I begin to use our mouths and tongues all over your cock. You can feel two mouths and two tongues moving all over your aching penis and balls, exploring every inch. You can feel hot breath on the sensitive, silky smooth skin of your shaft, and you don't know if it's mine or the prostitute's.

You clutch at our heads as we keep working on you. Your groin has never felt so good or so alive. You love the idea of two women working and sucking so hard on you. You've always fantasized about how it would feel, and now it's happening. You feel your cock slip past soft lips and down the back of a throat. You feel warm lips and tongues kissing and licking your scrotum. We're taking turns sucking on you. The head of your cock pushes past tight lips, first into my mouth, and then into the prostitute's. You're ready to explode, and I can see the bulging veins on your shaft.

You're doing the work of two, so suck, lick, pull, stroke, and kiss with sexual abandon. If he is really enjoying this, let him come.

Much of what you will describe as happening in this threesome is dependent on you and your partner's particular tastes. If he likes the idea of watching his woman and another woman perform oral sex or other sexual acts on each other, then incorporate that into the fantasy. You can have the prostitute and you perform oral sex on each other, fondle each other's breasts, and insert a finger into each other's vagina.

However, chances are good that your partner will prefer to

be the sole recipient of pleasure. If he has two women in his bed, even in his mind, he may want all the attention for himself! He's already imagined two women performing oral sex on him, and if he didn't come then, you can now add intercourse.

The prostitute and I stop sucking on you and kneel on either side of your body. You're exhausted. Your hard-on is so huge that you don't want to move...you just want release, and you need to come right away. You lie on the bed and look up at the two naked women leaning over you. You just lie there and wait, hoping that one of us will fuck you soon and give you relief from your pounding erection.

Kneel on the bed beside your man and run your fingers all over his body. Let him wait for it. After a few moments, straddle him. Position yourself over his penis and begin to lower yourself onto it. You're going to do all the work.

I instruct the prostitute to squat on top of you with her drenched pussy over your cock. I tell you that I'm going to let you come inside another woman while I watch. I tell you to lie still and enjoy the feeling of another woman's mound wrap around you. I push the prostitute's body down slowly onto your stiffness and you feel a surge of warmth as you enter her. I tell her to start fucking you.

Move cautiously up and down on your partner's penis, as if you are becoming accustomed to its size. Gradually, go as fast and hard as you and he like.

The prostitute moves herself up and down your shaft. She goes slowly at first, getting used to your penis inside her. Soon she's bouncing up and down vigorously. You close your eyes and lose yourself in the feeling of the prostitute's pussy hitting your body, and your cock plunging deep inside her. She's going at it so hard that the bed is shaking.

Tell your partner to grab your breasts.

You open your eyes and stare up at her body. Her large breasts are bouncing, and you reach up and grab them. They're soft and full in your hands. It's so strange to look up and see another woman's body on top of you, fucking you. It's mind-blowing to think that your cock is inside another woman's pussy right now.

Again you look up...I'm pushing down on the prostitute's shoulders to make her come down harder on you. I'm helping you fuck her. I tell you to shove it up inside her as far and as hard as you can. I want you to enjoy this as much as possible. I tell you to fuck her as long as you want, since that's what I'm paying her for. Soon you feel your orgasm building. You're desperate to feel the come erupt out of you. You need to feel that release. You grab the woman's waist, and both of us slam her body down onto your cock as hard as we can.

Move your man's hands to your waist and continue to move yourself up and down on him until both of you come. Do this eagerly and with lots of force and energy. You want him to become completely immersed in the fantasy. He should be frantically pushing himself up into you, totally lost in his desire, and thinking only of ejaculating into this prostitute in his own bedroom.

I tell you to come and you obey. The orgasm cripples you with pleasure and you look at me while you come inside the prostitute. She knows you're coming and she grinds herself onto you even harder. She lets you recover for a moment, then climbs off you.

Her work finished, the prostitute gets up and gets dressed. Businesslike, she takes the money off our nightstand and leaves. We watch her go, then lie back on the bed, just the two of us again. I whisper "Happy Birthday" into your ear, and as we race to the fridge for some leftover cake, you daringly remind me that my birthday is just around the corner.

AFTERWARD, tell your partner how much fun you had taking him through this fantasy. But tell him not to get too excited about his next birthday, since some things are better left to the imagination. For fun, have a surprise birthday cake or decorated cupcakes in the fridge to bring to bed after you've finished. It doesn't have to be his birthday for him to enjoy a sweet after sex. If you're feeling really generous, have a wrapped gift for him. Put some thought into it and buy something he's been wanting. Don't you love getting a surprise gift for no reason, other than the fact that you are loved and appreciated? And remember that the smile on your man's face as the party winds down is for you, not for any prostitute, however skilled she may be.

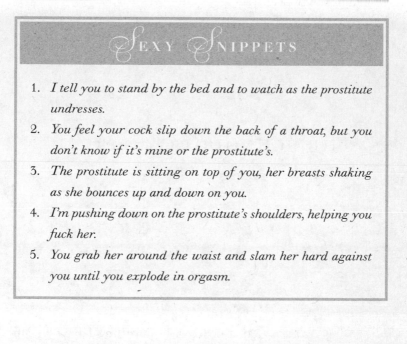

SEXY SNIPPETS

1. *I tell you to stand by the bed and to watch as the prostitute undresses.*

2. *You feel your cock slip down the back of a throat, but you don't know if it's mine or the prostitute's.*

3. *The prostitute is sitting on top of you, her breasts shaking as she bounces up and down on you.*

4. *I'm pushing down on the prostitute's shoulders, helping you fuck her.*

5. *You grab her around the waist and slam her hard against you until you explode in orgasm.*

11

THE SCHOOLGIRL AMBUSH

*M*ALE SEXUALITY can be baffling. I have yet to meet a man who doesn't admit to being sexually smitten by the schoolgirl uniform. On the one hand they like garter belts and push-up bras, and on the other they like white cotton panties and knee-high stockings. Why fight it? The schoolgirl uniform screams youthful innocence and is very off-limits, and many men seem to be incredibly turned on by this. In this fantasy, your partner finds himself straying into a sexual ambush set up by a group of lustful schoolgirls.

A bonus of this fantasy is that the schoolgirl uniform is so damn cute that just about anybody can look adorable in it. So, it's up to you whether you want to dress the part or just whisper the details into your man's ear and let his imagination do the rest. Whatever route you choose, expect to return to this fantasy again and again.

If you decide to dress the part, you'll need a short plaid

skirt, a white cotton shirt, dark blue knee-high stockings, black shoes, and a tie. Wear a simple white bra and white cotton panties underneath. Put your hair in pigtails or a ponytail if it's long enough. If it's not long enough, try just using a headband. Go easy on the makeup—shiny lip gloss that tastes like watermelon or bubblegum will do nicely. You can greet your partner at the door wearing this uniform, or change into it before coming to bed.

If you choose to simply whisper this fantasy in your man's ear and let his imagination dress it up, you must make sure that he has a clear picture of the schoolgirls and the schoolgirl uniform in his head so that he can really visualize what's going on. Wait until you're both in bed and snuggled up to each other.

You can ease into this fantasy by saying something like:

I overheard some guys talking at work today… one guy was telling the others how his neighbor's daughter just started attending this private all-girl college in town. He kept going on about her school uniform. He said he watches her through his kitchen every single morning as she leaves her house. What is it about those uniforms that turns men on so much?

As always, adopt a teasing tone of voice so that your partner knows it's okay for him to let his mind wander in this direction. Give him a picture of what you want him to see. Maybe he will want to respond, to tell you just what it is about those schoolgirls. If you want, ask him to lie on his stomach, and give him a backrub while you tell your story.

Can you picture one of those uniforms? There's a girl wearing a white cotton long-sleeved shirt and a short plaid skirt. She has dark knee-high stockings on, and shiny black shoes. There's a loosened school tie around her neck. She's also undone the top button of her shirt. The only makeup she's wearing is some shiny lip gloss that makes her lips look wet and pouting. Do you like what you see?

Now that your partner has a visual, begin to lead him through the plot of this fantasy. You must provide him with enough story, including physical and sensory details, to make the fantasy real to him.

Imagine that you're a worker, maybe an electrician or a maintenance man, and you've been called by this private college for girls to come and check some lights in the basement of the school. You're walking down a creaking old wood staircase into the dusty basement when you hear some muffled giggling behind a door.

You walk up to the door and notice that it's slightly ajar. You look at the number on the door and realize it's the room you were looking for in order to check some lights. You push the door open, and enter. It's only half-lit in the room, and it smells dank and old. It's a world away from the brightly lit and sterile schoolrooms upstairs. As your eyes are still adjusting, the door closes behind you.

Stroke your partner gently all over his body as you tell him this fantasy. He should be very relaxed and feel free to picture himself as the unsuspecting worker caught in the naughty schoolgirl trap. Tell him to close his eyes and imagine himself there. For a while you'll just be relating the details of this erotic story to him, letting him become aroused by the thought of it. Remember that sexual storytelling is verbal foreplay and should never be hurried.

You turn and look toward the closed door. There's a girl leaning against it, grinning. She's wearing her school uniform and looking very mischievous. She giggles, and all of a sudden three other schoolgirls emerge from their hiding spots behind some old bookshelves at the back of the room. The girls smile at one another and stare at you.

The girls seem shy but excited. One of them says, "We heard a man was coming by today to fix the lights down here. You don't mind if we watch you work, do you?" You tell them you don't mind, if they can tell you where to find a ladder.

As you work, the girls gather around the bottom of the ladder. You can hear them giggling and whispering things to each other. You're torn between just thinking they're cute and actually being turned on. You glance down and see one of the girls loosen her tie and undo some of the buttons on her shirt. From your vantage point you can see she's wearing a simple white bra, and you can just make out the curves of her breasts. They're bigger than they looked with her shirt done up.

Adjust yourself and the covers so that your man can just make out the curves of your breasts. Let yourself escape into the fantasy world too. Just as your partner is imagining himself as this workman, imagine yourself as one of these mischievous, frisky girls. Enjoy feeling naughty, and revel in the role of the "bad girl."

You climb down the ladder, and as you step off of it the girl brushes against you. Her breasts press into you and you can feel the soft flesh against your coveralls. She says a feigned "Oh, excuse me," and the other girls laugh. "We hang out lots down here," one of the girls tells you. "The school matron doesn't know we're down here, you know," says another.

Press your breasts against your partner's body, teasing him.

The girls circle around you. They're standing so close and smiling in a way that makes you think they're teasing you. They're definitely not as conservative as the school or their uniforms would like people to think.

Another girl says, "This is an all-girl school, you know ... and sometimes a girl has to take charge of her own education. Do you think you could help us with that? It's a little embarrassing to ask, but we really want to know." "Sure," you answer, you'll help them however you can.

The girls dart glances at one another. They all focus on one girl and whisper, "You ask him." The elected girl—you guess she's the bravest of the bunch—says, "We've only seen a man's body in our biology books. And that's just a drawing. Most girls our age have lots of experience with guys, but when you attend an all-girl school you're a bit sheltered. Do you think you could show us your ... ummm ... you know."

Move your hands down and caress your man's penis and testicles lightly. You want him to feel like his genitals are the center of everyone's attention—inside and outside the fantasy world.

The girls wait for you to answer. You can't believe they've asked you, and you know if you get caught you'll lose your job and your girlfriend. But they're so insistent and so innocent that you can't help yourself. They promise you that nobody else ever comes down to the basement and that there's no way anyone could catch you. And they won't tell anyone, they just want to see what a real man looks like. You can feel you're getting hard, and you wonder if they know the difference between an erect and non-erect cock.

You can tell the girls are getting excited too. One of them brushes her hands over her nipples, then bites her lip and looks

*at the floor. You even think you see one of them touching her-
self.*

Begin to touch yourself, doing what feels good. Slip your
fingers under your top to touch your breasts, then under your
panties to feel between your legs.

*You're wondering what to say and do when one of the girls
says, "If we take our clothes off, will you take off yours?" You
know you should say no. You know you should run out of there
and not look back, but your cock pounds at the thought of these
naked girls looking at you, the first naked man they've ever
seen. Everything in your mind is telling you to leave, but your
body betrays you and you can't move. You can't say no. You're
so filled with desire that you don't trust yourself.*

*One of the girls starts to unbutton her shirt, and you can't
pull your eyes away. She opens her shirt all the way and pulls
the tie off over her head without taking her eyes off you. The
other girls follow her example, filling the room with the rustle
of shirts dropping to the floor. Before you know it, you're surrounded by all four of the girls wearing their bras. Then, one
by one, they remove their bras, exposing their bare breasts,
their taut nipples.*

Remove your top and bra completely, letting your partner
enjoy the sight of your own breasts. Trace your nipples with
a wet finger. Ask your partner if he'd like to try—but then
continue with the fantasy.

*Their nipples are pink and hard, and although you don't
know if it's from the cold or the excitement, you get harder anyway.*

*One of the girls says to the others, "Take off your skirts or he
won't do it." They all push their short skirts to the floor and*

*step out of them. They peel off their stockings and stand before
you wearing only little panties.*

This might be a good moment to remove your remaining
clothes. Be coy, girlish, and play the schoolgirl part. Leave
only your panties on.

*The girl who just spoke comes closer to you. Her breasts are
small, the nipples tight, and you have an uncontrollable urge to
reach out and touch them. You risk it, and as soon as your hand
touches her flesh she gasps, but doesn't move away.*

Take your man's hand and guide it to your breasts, making
him feel and caress them. Take one of his fingertips, get it
wet in your mouth, and trace your nipple with it. Show him
the rush of pleasure you experience as his hand caresses you.

*The girl smiles and bites her bottom lip. She looks at you
mischievously, waiting for you to give her that sensation again.
You cup both her breasts in your hands and she leans her head
back in ecstasy. The other girls are wide-eyed for a moment, but
then begin to caress their own breasts. You can tell they wonder
what it feels like to be touched by a man like that.*

*You unzip your work coveralls and take off your shirt and
pants as fast as you can. You stand in front of them wearing just
your briefs, and all their eyes are glued on your dick poking at
the fabric. They can't wait to see what it looks like.*

Undress your partner with hurried desperation, as if you're
anxious to see his penis. Get into the role by pretending you've
never seen it before, and can't wait.

*As you remove your shorts, your cock springs up completely
erect and incredibly hard. You can see the girls parting and
licking their lips at the sight of it. One by one they approach
you.*

You know that in just a moment one or maybe all of the girls

will reach out and you'll feel her soft hands caress your hard-
ness. One of them says, "He has hair, just like us." You look
down and see eight soft hands moving all over the shaft and
head of your cock. It's everything you can do not to come right
then and there. The girls are marveling at your body. They
can't believe how hard or how big a man can get. But they're not
just touching you there. They're running their hands over your
ass, your thighs, your chest. One of them steps back, as if she
wants a better view.

Touch your partner's penis with curious and exploring
hands, but don't stop there. Get his whole body involved.

One of the girls asks you what a blow job is. She wants to
know if you're really supposed to blow, or what? You tell her
that she's only supposed to suck it, and she asks if she can see
what it feels like. You nod and she kneels in front of you. For a
moment all you feel is her hot breath on your shaft, but soon
you feel her moist lips wrap uncertainly around it.

Kneel between your man's spread legs. Breathe onto his
penis, and then wrap your lips around it. Perform oral sex
with amateurish enthusiasm.

You can tell she's never done this before since she doesn't have
any real technique. But that doesn't matter. Just the thought of
this inexperienced girl sucking on you and having your cock in
her mouth is enough to keep you stimulated. Your eyes are
squeezed shut with the pleasure of it, and you hardly notice that
each of the girls is taking turns practicing on you.

Continue performing oral sex on your partner as long as
you like. If you want him to come like this, let him.

If you're in the mood for intercourse, begin like this:

Through the overwhelming stimulation centered in your
groin, you hear one of the girls say to the others, "So who

wants to do it?" You keep your eyes closed, abandoning yourself to what is happening. There's no way in the world you could stop yourself now. If one of these girls offers herself to you, you'll fuck her in an instant, no matter what the consequences are.

You've never felt blood racing through your body or to your dick like this before. You can't remember ever being so painfully hard.

Stop performing oral sex. Still kneeling between your partner's spread legs, lean over him and stroke his thighs as you continue relating the story.

Your cock is throbbing hard and your heart is pounding loudly. You hear a shaky voice say, "Could you show us how it goes into a girl?" You nod because you can't find your voice.

The girl then asks you to pick which one of them you'd like to demonstrate on. You look at them. They're all young and pretty, and you choose the one you think is prettiest. The girl smiles and asks, "What should I do?" You direct her to lie down on the floor, and you tell the other girls to watch. You kneel down beside her and pull down her white cotton panties.

Lie down flat and have your man pull your panties off. Squirm out of them anxiously.

Imagine this naked girl lying right underneath you, waiting to feel a man enter her for the first time. Standing all around, watching, there are three other naked girls who wish you were doing it to them instead. They're imagining that they're the one lying under you and feeling your body on top of them.

You get in the missionary position and reach your hand down between the girl's legs. She's dripping with wetness and anticipation, and when she feels your hand down there her whole body shudders.

Pull your partner on top of you in the missionary position. Direct him to take his penis and rub the head against your vagina. Spread your legs wide, showing him the pleasure you feel.

You place the sensitive head of your cock at the very opening of her pussy and she reflexively spreads her legs wide open for you. You push yourself inside her... she's really tight, and you have to steady yourself and push harder. Finally your swollen cock sinks deep inside her. At first she gasps, then gradually her pain turns into a new, intense pleasure and she begins to moan.

When your man enters you, make like it's the first time; act a little afraid, offer some resistance, and pretend that it hurts. He may be thrilled by this unexpected reaction from you. Act like the inexperienced schoolgirl throughout your lovemaking. It will heighten the pleasure for both of you.

She wraps her legs around you and tries to meet your thrusts, although she's so inexperienced that she can't really match your rhythm. You can feel the eyes of the other girls on your naked ass and back as, from above, they watch you having sex, thrusting in and out of their friend. Suddenly the girl screams and claws wildly at your back. She's having her first orgasm, and you almost have to hold her down to keep your cock in her.

When you reach orgasm, make the most of it. Allow yourself to react dramatically as it washes over you. Again, this response will make the feeling more raw and intense for both of you.

To bring your partner to orgasm, reassert the visual of what is happening to him.

Imagine yourself fucking this girl in the basement of this school, with her friends standing around you and watching you on the floor. You're making this girl come for the first time. Now you want her to feel the fullness of a man coming inside her pussy.

You come fast and hard, and the force of your orgasm throws your head back. You know the girl is surprised by the fluid she feels jetting inside her, since she gasps and grabs at your shoulders as her pussy fills with come. You keep thrusting until your orgasm subsides.

Your man should have no trouble coming while you are describing this scene. When you feel him coming, claw at his back and shoulders as if you are overwhelmed by the force of his orgasm. Your reaction will intensify his orgasm even more.

You look at the girl's face and see that she is smiling. You roll off of her, exhausted and exhilarated. She and her friends gather their clothes and dress quickly, giggling to each other. They tell you that you're their favorite teacher, but that they're late for their next class. As you hastily zip up your coveralls, they grin at you over their shoulders and slip out of the room. You peek out the door and watch them dart down the hall, their pleated skirts bouncing as they run up the stairs.

AFTERWARD, tell your man how much fun you had taking him through this fantasy, but inform him that the student bodies of all-girl schools aren't quite so innocent in the real world. And remember that the smile on his face as he recovers from this raw and intense fantasy is for you, his darling, generous woman, and not for the shameless schoolgirls.

SEXY SNIPPETS

1. *You're in the basement of this school and you can't take your eyes off these bad schoolgirls . . . their full young breasts and tight pussies are all around you.*

2. *You look down and see eight soft hands moving all over the shaft and head of your cock, exploring you.*

3. *One of the girls asks you what a blow job is, and whether she can try one on you.*

4. *You push your dick into her tight pussy. There's some resistance, but you ease it into her wet warmth.*

5. *You can feel the other girls watching as you fill their friend with come.*

12

THE CHEAP MOTEL

*M*Y HUSBAND used to travel a lot for work and consequently spent many nights alone in a stream of motels and hotels. The accommodations ranged from the dingiest motels to the finest hotels, depending on location and availability. He revealed to me that when he was staying at the less glamorous establishments, he often fantasized about the motel providing hookers for his pleasure, or about cruising through the unfamiliar town and picking up a local prostitute to bring back to his room.

He explained that it was the combination of anonymity and raunchiness that fueled this fantasy, and that it was an idea he often masturbated to when traveling. Many men love the idea of being "serviced," and there's no better or more natural place to fantasize about this than in a motel or hotel. In this fantasy, room service takes on a whole new meaning.

If you have the time and the inclination, arrange for your partner and you to stay in a cheap motel in your own city. It'll add spontaneity, fun, and realism to your fantasy. If not, this fantasy works just as well at home.

When you're tucked into bed with your partner, inquire shyly about scenarios he used to or still does masturbate to. He may be hesitant to reveal such personal details, but if you adopt a nonjudgmental and reassuring demeanor, he might actually enjoy telling all. To make it even easier for him, tell him thoughts you masturbate to.

The information your partner reveals will provide you with material to design your own stories to fulfill his personal fantasies, and the discussion itself will arouse him enough to provide an opening to this fantasy. You can ask him if any situation or location was or is particularly stimulating. He might even surprise you and say a motel.

If your man doesn't bite, reveal to him—whether it's true or not—that you find staying in a motel turns you on. Tell him that you remember staying in a seedy motel for some forgotten reason in the past, and that your loneliness got the better of you. Tell him that you remember thinking how incredibly erotic it would've been to spend the night in a dirty motel room with a complete stranger. Tell him that you masturbated at the thought of it. Chances are he'll be turned on just by picturing you in that situation.

You can say something like:

Everybody always says how good motel sex is. You're away from home, and nobody knows what you're doing or who you're doing it with. It's like you can be someone else. Have you ever stayed in a really seedy motel?

Set the stage for the fantasy so your partner can visualize himself in it. Speak in a naughty voice, and press your body against his. Show him your excitement.

Can you imagine yourself in a dirty, cramped little motel room? It's one of those where you drive your car right up to the door. The walls are paper thin, the room is dimly lit, and the bed and bedspreads are old and worn. There's a small television with an outdated remote control. The neon sign is flashing "Vacancy" and "XXX Movies," and the electric light pierces the sheer curtain to fill the room for a second, then fades away just as fast.

Continue by gradually introducing a storyline to the fantasy.

You're away from home, in a strange city, on a business trip. There were no other hotels in town so you had to come to this old motel in the dirty downtown area. It's a completely different world than the one you're accustomed to in suburbia with your wife and kids.

If you and your partner aren't married, no matter. It's up to you whether you want to pretend he is—either to you or to someone else—to emphasize the "cheating" aspect of this fantasy. Similarly, it doesn't matter whether or not you really have children. You can build these elements into the fantasy world and your partner's fantasy life, or you can just omit them altogether.

You drop your suitcases on the floor and sit on the edge of the bed. It's old and rickety and it squeaks as soon as your weight hits it. You can hear the muffled sounds in the rooms on either side of yours. From one side you can hear the din of the TV, and from the other the shower running. You can hear footsteps and voices filtering down from the room above you. You're lonely and, even with all the sounds in the motel, bored.

You begin to look for something to entertain you. You flick on the TV and blankly watch some commercials. You're lying on the cheap bedspread when you notice some pamphlets on the nightstand. You flip through them. Most of them are from pizza parlors, but one of them catches your eye.

The pamphlet has the words "Need a date tonight?" and "Only you and I need to know" printed on thin pink paper. It has an amateurish graphic of a woman's lips pursed in a kiss. There's also a silhouette of a woman's breasts and a phone number. You throw it on the floor and try to forget about it.

Rather than simply describing this pamphlet to your partner, you might want to take the time to create it. This is easily enough done on any computer, and you can jazz it up any way you like. Draw or print whatever you think will arouse your partner the most. We all know that a picture is worth a thousand words. In fact, you may want to simply hand this pamphlet to him when you first crawl into bed, and start the fantasy from there. He won't be expecting to see something like that in his own bedroom, and just the sight of it may stimulate him. Best of all, it's a fun and playful thing to do, and will help both of you relax and get into the fantasy.

Continue with the story.

You're just lying on the bed, channel surfing. It's getting close to midnight but you're not tired enough to go to sleep yet. You're flipping through the channels when suddenly you come across some porn...the stark image of naked bodies appears on the screen and surprises you. You stay on this channel. There's a woman sandwiched between two men. She's lying on top of one and the other is lying on top of her. She's giving a third man a blow job.

You try to figure out exactly what they're doing and find that you're a little turned on when you realize that all the men have their cocks inside her. The one on the bottom is in her pussy and the one on top is in her ass. The third man is in her mouth. They're all fucking her at the same time, and she's in such ecstasy that she looks drunk.

Now that you've introduced this erotic scene into the fantasy, add physical stimulation to your man's mental arousal by running your fingers lightly and teasingly over his skin. Don't touch his genitals just yet.

You can feel your pulse quicken immediately and involuntarily in response. Your cock begins to throb and you recognize the familiar dull ache that rises and then settles in your groin.

You know you should change channels. You don't want to get too turned on, since there's nothing you can do about it. You're used to having your wife's body, so masturbating isn't as satisfying as it used to be when you were single. You like the real thing. But you can't stop watching the screen.

The man on top climbs off the woman. He takes his dick in his hand and brings it close to the woman's mouth. You can see the come stream out of it and all over her face. You start thinking about how good it feels to come and how wonderful that release would feel right now. You're touching yourself and you're getting hard.

Now take your partner's hand and direct it toward his penis. Rub him lightly with your hands and with his.

You're staring at the TV when a certain sound begins to creep into your consciousness. You realize that, for some time now, the sound of this same channel has been drifting down from the room above. You realize the people upstairs are watch-ing the same thing you are. You lower the volume and listen more closely. Sure enough, you hear the bed above squeaking and squeaking in a smooth, regular rhythm.

As this idea enters your man's mind, begin to touch his pe-nis with more pressure and urgency. This will complement the increasing steaminess of the fantasy.

You wish that your wife's body were next to you so you could just crawl on top of her and satisfy yourself. The dirtiness of the room and the sounds above you start to crowd your mind with things that ordinarily you would never consider even for a mo-ment. You start to think about the pamphlet and the possibilities it offers. You're getting weak and you know it... but you can't help yourself.

You pick the pamphlet up off the floor. Again you read the words "Need a date tonight?" and "Only you and I need to know." You think about how lucky the guy upstairs is, and how much you wish you were him right now. Your desire is building by the second and you know you're going to have to satisfy it somehow. You think again about masturbating, but you want more. You want to feel a woman's breasts and skin pressing against your skin. You want to feel hands over your body.

You start to think about how different it would be to touch another woman... you've been married a long time. You love your wife, but right now you can't help but think about fucking a total stranger, no strings attached. Almost against your will, you pick up the phone and dial the number on the pamphlet.

Reassure your partner that it's okay for him to enjoy these thoughts. Almost all men will at one time or another think about another woman, so let him think about an imaginary woman in this fun and unthreatening way.

A woman answers the phone. Her voice is throaty. She asks,
"Are you looking for company tonight?" You manage to stutter,
"Yes, I think so. I'm from out of town. I'm staying at the Lucky
Star Motel…um, how does this, um…" The woman breaks in
and says, "Lots of our girls visit gentlemen at the Lucky Star,
don't you worry. Why don't you tell me what kind of girl you'd
like to spend some time with?"

You stare back at the TV and look at the porn star. She has a
bad bleach job with dark streaks, and big, pouting red lips. She's
on her hands and knees and a man is fucking her from behind.
He's pounding into her really hard and her huge breasts are
shaking back and forth.

You describe the porn star to the woman on the phone. She
asks for your room number and tells you the girls accept only
cash. She tells you someone will be there by 12:30 A.M. You hang
up the phone and look at the clock. It's just after midnight. You
can feel your cock get harder with anticipation as each minute
passes.

Take a break from the storyline to ask your man what he
thinks it would be like to be in that little dingy room waiting
for a hooker to show up at the door. Ask him what he might
be thinking. Would he be nervous? Regretful? Or would he be
so anxious for her to show up that the wait would be agony?

After about twenty minutes you see a shadow move past your
window and there's a knock at the door. You get off the bed and
walk toward the door. Your dick is uncomfortably hard now,
and the friction from your tight jeans makes it stiffen and ache.
You can't believe you're doing this. It's like you're in a movie or
something, and that's how you're imagining yourself right
now. If you really thought about the reality of your situation
you'd never go through with it, but your desire is blinding you

to reality. You feel like you're on automatic pilot, and that your need for sexual release is in control of your body and your choices.

You're aware of your nervousness, and of how wrong it is to be going through with this. You open the door anyway. You're more desperate than embarrassed. A woman that looks remarkably similar to the porn star smiles at you and brushes past you into the room without saying a word. You shut the door behind you. The walls seem to close in on you and this hooker in the small, dark room.

You feel like you're someone else completely. Your former life doesn't even exist. You're just this guy in a cheap motel room who hired a hooker to get off. The hooker turns and looks at you, sizing you up. Images of all the dirty things she must have done flash through your mind and make your penis throb in your jeans. She looks down at the growing bulge in your pants and licks her moist lips.

Be sure to imagine yourself as this hooker. Imagine all the things she's done, and all the things she's seen. Allow yourself to give in to the dirtiness and the freedom, and to think about sex in this way. These fantasies are as much for you to experience sex in a different way, and from a different perspective, as they are for your partner to do so.

"I'm glad you wanted company tonight ... there's no reason for a man like you to sit in a motel room all alone." She glances up at the television and watches the porn for a few moments. "That looks like fun, don't you think?" She motions to the screen and you look up. The woman is now sitting on top of one of the men and giving the other two hand jobs.

The sounds from the television fill the room, mesmerizing you. The hooker tells you how much it'll cost you, and you nod in agreement. You can't believe you're going to give a woman money to have sex with you, and you're surprisingly aroused by the idea of paying for it.

Continue to touch your partner's genitals. Squeeze his penis and rub your palm over the head. Squeeze his testicles and tickle his perineum. Stroke the inside of his thighs, and move your hands all over his body.

The hooker steps toward you and the bed, and you get a closer look at her. She's wearing tight blue jeans with high boots and a fake black leather jacket. She's moderately attractive, but a little rough around the edges. She's pretty much what you'd expect to find in a place like this, and she fits in well with the surroundings. The fact that she's as dirty as the motel turns you on. You figure that if you're going to have dirty sex in a motel, you might as well get the most out of it.

The hooker seems to read your mind and says, "Now's your chance to do all the things you've always wanted to try . . . I'll do whatever you ask. I'll do what your woman won't. You can do anything you want to my body and I'll do whatever you want to yours. Nothing is off-limits tonight."

Adopt the language you imagine a hooker would use. It may be difficult at first, but at least give it a try to see if you like it. Talking dirty turns many men and women on, but the degree and specifics are up to you. Use words that you and your partner find arousing, and that you are comfortable with. That being said, don't be afraid to summon the courage to experiment by going a little further. You never know unless you try. Even if you overstep the bounds of what you consider good taste, it'll give you both a laugh.

It's now time to ask for your partner's input. It's essential that you make him realize he can tell you his dirtiest and most taboo sexual thoughts and desires.

The hooker will do absolutely anything you want her to. She'll suck you, let you come on her or in her—even let you fuck her in the ass. She's not your typical hooker. She tells you it's really tight. She says it's something most men secretly want to try, but don't want their partners to know.

Don't be afraid to say this. Even if your partner wants to explore anal sex and you don't, you can keep it in the realm of fantasy by just pretending.

The hooker starts to take her clothes off. You can tell by her matter-of-fact attitude that she's done this a thousand times. She takes off her jacket and steps out of her high boots. She pulls off her tight blue jeans and takes off her shirt. She's wearing red lace panties and a red lace bra that are faded and don't match exactly. You know she's a cheap hooker but that's perfect for tonight, in this place. Her breasts are so large that you know they're fake. They spill out the sides of the bra, almost falling out. Normally that would turn you off, but tonight it has the opposite effect.

Renew and revive your partner's visualization.

Imagine that you're standing by the bed in this cheap motel room, staring at this nearly naked hooker. Your groin is pounding with blood. The room is filled with flickering light from the television and the sounds of moaning coming from the porn on the screen.

Caress your man all over his body as you review the scene. Remember that the idea of where he is, and with whom, is what will arouse him, so you must make him imagine it is really happening to him.

You know you're going to come really fast. The idea of being with a hooker like this has made you so hard that you know you can't last much longer. You have to get relief from your hard-on. You take off your clothes as fast as you can. You're not embarrassed, or nervous, or anything . . . you just want to get off.

The hooker knows what's coming, and she knows you're ready to get down to business. She asks you how you want it. It's up to you. If you want, she'll tongue your ass so you can feel what it's like to have your anus stimulated. She tells you she'll do whatever you want. You just have to tell her how you want to come.

Let your partner decide what he wants to do to your body or have done to his. If he seems curious to have his own anus stimulated, don't hesitate to accommodate him unless you are really opposed. You can use your tongue and/or your finger to circle the outside of his anus. Gently insert a well-lubricated finger into his anus, pull out, and gauge his response. You will have to be the judge of how long you do this. If he starts to become flaccid, which he may if the experience is new, stop and use your mouth on his penis to rev him up again.

Let your partner decide how he wants to have you. If he chooses anal intercourse and that's okay with you, make sure that you use lots of lubrication and a condom, and relax your muscles. Tell him to go slow and not to thrust too hard. If at any time it becomes painful, stop! No fantasy is worth hurting yourself.

If you are unwilling to do anal sex, you can at least partly satisfy his desire for anal penetration by just pretending. Squeeze your hand tightly around his penis while he visualizes himself thrusting into the hooker's anus. Bear in mind that a vivid description of events is even more crucial if he is just using his imagination.

It feels so good in my ass... you've never had it like this before, have you? Imagine yourself fucking this hooker in the ass... it feels so tight and so different.

If your man wants to have a blow job from this hooker, give him one. If he wants to have you in a new or unusual position, let him. Anything goes, since the customer is always right. Make lots of noise during the experience—vary your moans and don't be afraid to let out a few screams or shrieks. If you sound different to him during the sexual experience, it will be much easier for him to imagine you are someone else. Similarly, change the way you normally move your body during sex. Grab and clutch at him in ways you don't usually do. Move aggressively and shamelessly, and let yourself come whenever the feeling strikes. This will help you to immerse yourself in your role and have the most fun possible.

To bring the fantasy to an end, let him come however he wants.

INSTEAD of having your partner imagine that he finds a pamphlet in his room, you can alternatively begin the fantasy by having him picture himself cruising up and down unfamiliar city streets, searching for a hooker to bring back to his motel room.

The idea of cruising for a hooker is a turn-on for many people. There's a certain sexual curiosity many of us share when it comes to streetwalkers, and few of us can stop ourselves from looking when driving past. Many men have seen hookers on the street corner, and it is naïve to think they haven't on occasion fantasized about picking one up. This makes for perfect fantasy material.

If you choose this second version for the start of this fantasy, you can bring up the idea of sex-for-money by saying something like:

I saw on the news there's a real problem with street prostitution at such-and-such a place. They showed pictures of these women hanging out on the corner and these cars slowing down . . . the women would go up to the cars and lean in the window, I'm assuming to negotiate terms. They were all dressed in really short tight skirts and high heels or boots.

You can then adopt a more teasing tone that will let your partner know you're ready to play.

You've seen those women on the street, I'm sure you've driven by them. Have you ever fantasized about actually picking one of them up? Have you ever slowed down to look at them? Have you ever been so desperate that you actually considered picking one up? Imagine yourself when you were single, maybe in the middle of a romantic dry spell. It's been months and months since you've been with a woman and you're feeling very neglected.

Set the scene and tell the tale.

You're out of town, on business or visiting some friends or something, and you're staying at a motel. You're driving back to your motel at night and you get lost. You end up in the sketchy part of town, and you start to notice girls standing along the street. You know they're prostitutes just by the way they're dressed and how they're walking down the street.

A couple of cars are pulled over ahead of you and there are women leaning into the windows, talking to the drivers. You imagine they're talking about how much money different things will cost. You watch as a tall redhead wearing a mini-skirt gets into one of the cars, and when the car takes off you're jealous. You wish you could be getting what that guy is about to get. You wonder if he's buying some quick head or something a little pricier.

You want to make your partner remember a time when he was so desperate for sexual contact that he did or would have considered picking up a hooker. Caress his skin with your fingertips while you describe this to him.

You start to think to yourself...you're out of town, nobody knows you, and it's been a long, long time. Too long. You've been away on business and it's been months since you had sex.

Drag your fingertips lightly over his forehead, then trace his jawline.

Picture yourself sitting in your car, late at night in a strange city, with prostitutes within reach. Your balls ache at the very idea of bringing one back to your motel room. It would be so easy to do with some money. All you have to do is stop the car, and they'll do the work. They'll approach and you can pick and choose which one you want to fuck. It's that easy. You have the money. Now you just need the nerve. The more you think about it, the more your groin responds. Finally you pull your car over a few yards from several women.

It only takes a minute before a woman walks up to your car and leans into the window. She's blonde, wearing tight jeans and a black fake leather jacket. She's rough around the edges, but she'll do whatever you have in mind. You don't care, you just want a body to fuck.

Take a break from the storyline to ask your partner if he

would ever really hire a hooker, and, if he has, what pushed him to do it. Ask him what he'd have a hooker do if she was straddling his lap right now. Then continue on.

You're getting so hard while this girl tells you how much she costs. She tells you how much a blow job will set you back, how much for a missionary-style fuck—and how much for in the ass. She tells you that she can do it in your car, or you two can go somewhere. It's up to you and it's that simple. She waits for you to answer.

You can't believe the words are coming out of your mouth, but you tell her to get in. It's almost surreal. Your dick is fighting against your jeans. You imagine how good it will feel to unzip your pants and let it burst out. You imagine how good it will feel when this hooker finally sucks it or sticks it in her, or whatever you're going to make her do.

Sure, it's not the language you're used to, but you're in the bedroom, not the boardroom. And it'll add to the sense of growing desperation you both should be feeling.

The hooker gets in the passenger door of your car and you drive back to the motel. She's so close that it's dizzying. Her cheap perfume fills the interior of the car. It smells like sex. The closer you get to the motel, the harder you get. You pull up to the door of your room and both of you go inside without saying a word.

You can now pick up the fantasy from where your partner and the hooker are in the motel room together.

AFTERWARD, let your partner know how much fun you had. Let him know how much you value the trust and friendship in your relationship, and how happy you are to be the woman leading him through these fantasies. As always, tell him what a great lover he is, and how sexy he makes you feel. Give him a receipt or slip of paper that you took the liberty of hiding under your bed, and share a laugh as you fill it out for services rendered. Make sure your man feels comfortable afterward. He'll follow your lead, so take care never to make him feel embarrassed or guilty. And remember that the smile on his face is for you, not for the motel guest.

Sexy Snippets

1. *You've never wanted another body so badly. You imagine how good it would feel to sink your dick into a warm, wet pussy, one you haven't felt before.*
2. *You can hear sucking sounds from the porn on TV as the hooker begins to suck your cock.*
3. *She'll let you do anything . . . you can fuck her in the mouth or in the ass, whatever you like.*
4. *Her breasts are large and feel wonderful under your hands.*
5. *The hooker is getting off. She loves it when she gets a cock like yours.*

13

THE FRENCH MAID

Ah oui, the French maid. The classic male sexual fantasy.

Like the Cheap Motel fantasy, the French Maid fantasy exploits the sense of sexual freedom and anonymity that comes with being a stranger in a strange town. But an extra erotic element is added to the mix in this fantasy, which is set in a five-star hotel: specifically, a sinful temptress dressed in a little white apron and fishnet stockings.

The French Maid fantasy is so popular that any self-respecting costume shop will be able to supply you with a uniform, should you wish to fully dress the part. It's up to you how deeply you want to dive into the role-play. You can spring a sexy surprise on your partner by wearing high stockings and a garter under your usual clothes, or you can forgo the wardrobe work and simply whisper the dialogue into his ear as you make love—in a lustful French accent, of course.

If you have the time and the resources, arrange to stay at the most elegant posh hotel that your city has to offer. Make sure it has a jet tub. This will provide the perfect setting to play out this frisky favorite, and it will add spontaneity, fun, and luxurious realism to your fantasy. (There's no reason you have to leave town to have a vacation.) However, this fantasy works just as well in your own bedroom.

Just as you do every fantasy night, make sure that you are shower-fresh, your skin is soft, smooth, and scented, and that you are wearing some tasty lip gloss when you get into bed with your partner. Leave a bedside light on in the room, since you'll need a bit of light to enjoy this fantasy to the fullest.

If you are at home, it would be a helpful complement to this fantasy to put some brand-new crisp white sheets on your bed. Use the type they use in expensive hotels to appeal to your partner's senses and help transport his mind. You could even prewash them in a different-scented detergent to further distance both of you to the feel and smell of your normal bed. As always, it's up to you how much time and effort you want to invest in fantasy night. Do as much as necessary to put yourself in the mood so you enjoy it as much as possible.

When you're both tucked in and ready for some pillow talk, say something to the effect of:

Did you notice the new sheets I bought? I feel like I'm sleeping in a hotel bed! That reminds me ... I saw this advertisement today for the most gorgeous hotel I've ever seen.

You'll have to fabricate a little.

It's in [name the city], and it's probably the ritziest one in town. Definitely a five-star. The room they showed had a huge, king-size bed with these big cherrywood bedposts. It was just gorgeous. There was a jet tub right beside the bed so you could step directly out of the tub and jump into bed! And right beside the tub, basically out in the open, was a stall-type shower. It was really different, but beautiful. It must cost a fortune. I was thinking how wonderful it would be to stay there—with you, of course. It wouldn't be any fun to stay there alone, would it?

Slip into fantasy mode and set the scene for your partner.

Can you picture yourself in a hotel like that, all alone? No one to share it with. What a waste! Imagine that you are in another city on business, and your wife is at home, hundreds of miles away.

Unlike the Cheap Motel fantasy, the storyline here requires that your partner be married in the fantasy world, whether to you or to someone else.

Give your partner the usual indicators that you're about to take him on a little trip. When he's relaxed and comfortable enough to let his mind drift and his desire mount, continue to set up the fantasy for him.

Imagine that it's late at night and you've just checked in to this very expensive hotel. You open the door to an exquisite room and toss your bags in the corner. You eye the jet tub and wish that your wife were there to share it with you. It's been days and days since you've had any intimate physical contact, and you're really starting to long for it. You think about how incredible it would feel right now to be naked in the water with another naked body to press up against.

You take off your shoes and start to wind down. You turn on the stereo and some soft, relaxing music fills the strange room. You're so tired and so relaxed that you don't have a worry in the world right now.

Make your partner as relaxed as possible. Run your hands over his body, and tell him to take some deep breaths and let himself melt into the bed. Maybe take some massage oil to rub into and warm his skin while you lead him into the fantasy.

You've been in the same clothes since very early in the morning, so you decide to take a quick shower before climbing between those clean, crisp white sheets—just like the ones you're lying on now. You strip by the bed and then walk across the room completely naked.

It feels strangely liberating to be walking naked in this elaborate hotel room. The plush carpet on your feet is like a foot massage, and the warm room air feels wonderful against your bare skin. You feel very exposed as you step into the shower in the middle of the room, but you kind of like the feeling. The warm water cascades over your skin and you can feel all your stress and worries washing away.

Your partner should be able to see—in his mind's eye—the shower, the jet tub, the bed with the crisp white sheets, and the plush carpet. He should be able to feel the liberating sense of naked exposure, the warm water running down his back, and the dissolution of his stress and worries. Your goal is to turn this and every fantasy into a sensual mini mind-and-body vacation for you and your partner.

You turn off the water and open the shower door. You reach for a towel and step out of the shower, still dripping wet. All of a sudden you have the sense that you're not alone, and you look up to find a hotel chambermaid staring back at you.

The maid is as surprised to see you as you are to see her. She looks embarrassed, but doesn't look away. She apologizes in an adorable French accent and says that she was just trying to slip in quickly and stock your room with some fresh towels. You're just standing there, naked and dripping water, and she's just staring at your body.

The maid takes a step toward you, takes a towel, and hands it to you. For some reason you don't cover yourself with it right away. You like the feeling of her looking at you. Finally, almost regretfully, you accept the towel and wrap it around your waist. Your testicles contract, and the friction from the cotton towel feels good pressed against you.

Touch your partner's testicles lightly with your fingertips. Tease them a little, and gently massage the perineum.

Instead of excusing herself, the maid lingers. She asks you if there's anything you or your room needs, and for the first time you take a good look at her. She's wearing a tiny black skirt that barely covers her ass, and you catch a glimpse of the garter belt holding up her high stockings. A small white apron is tied tightly around her slight waist, showing off her hourglass figure even more. Her black hair is pulled back in a tight bun. She looks to be thirty-something and she's beautiful. Her lips are very full, almost like she's had some work done to them. Your wife would probably laugh and call them "porn lips," and you smile to yourself at the thought.

But your wife is hundreds of miles and another world away right now. Your real life seems like a whole other reality to you at this moment, completely removed from what's going on in this hotel room. The maid says she's going to prepare your bed for you. She walks over to the bed and pulls back the downy comforter to reveal the snow-white sheets.

Just as your partner should be immersed in his role as the lonely husband on a business trip, so should you immerse yourself in your role as the tempting, seductive French maid. Use your best French accent, or at least try speaking in broken English. Adopt a naughty tone and body language, as you show your admiration for this gorgeous guest as he steps, naked and dripping wet, out of the shower.

The maid asks you if you'd like her to run the jet tub for you. Her accent lends her voice a foreign, velvety feel that you find very sensual. She tells you it would be a shame not to take advantage of the room's facilities. You've completely forgotten how tired you were, and you're suddenly very awake and alive. You say, "Sure, thanks," and walk over to the tub. You start to wonder what, if anything, you should wear into the tub ... your underwear? That would look silly, she's already seen you naked.

The maid bends over directly in front of you and starts to fill the tub. Her heart-shaped ass sticks up and you feel the urge to reach out and touch it. You get another glimpse of the garter under her short skirt, and if she bent down just a little more you would be able to see her panties. You have a fleeting visual of your cock entering her from behind, and the image stiffens you up.

Caress your partner's penis with light, teasing strokes. Make tiny circles on the frenulum with your fingertips, and tap the head very gently. Vary your touches so his penis feels a variety of sensations.

When the tub is full the maid turns to you and tells you to get in. She reaches out and casually pulls the towel off of you, asking if there's anything else she can get for you. You shake your head and step quickly into the tub, hoping she won't notice your growing erection. The water is hot, almost too hot, and you can feel the jets of water stroking your back. It feels great. You lean back and take a deep breath. For the first time you notice there is a very large mirror on the wall beside the tub. You gaze into it.

As if in a daze, you stare at yourself, but you can hardly recognize the naked man in the tub. Through the mirror, you can see the maid busying herself with the towels behind you. She's stalling for time and you know it. For some reason she wants to stay in the room with you. You wonder if she's thinking sexually, and you can't think of any other reason for her behavior. You put your head back, close your eyes, and enjoy the idea that she is thinking about you.

If you already have a large mirror in your bedroom, great. If not, consider introducing one. The bigger, the better. You can have it under the bed and pull it out at this point in the fantasy; this will give you both a good laugh, and will excite your partner as he realizes he is about to watch the two of you having sex. If you don't want to interrupt the story, have the mirror out when you get into bed. Its presence will immediately make your partner anticipate a fun night.

Sit up, have your partner sit up, and begin to massage his shoulders. Tell him to watch in the mirror and to imagine it is steamy from the heat of the tub.

Your thoughts are unexpectedly interrupted by a jolt of sensation as you feel hands on your shoulders. The maid is rubbing them. You open your eyes slowly, turn your head, and gaze again into the mirror beside the tub. The scene is like one from a movie. There's steam on the mirror from the hot bath, and that makes what you see even more sensual. You look at the maid's face in the mirror and see that she's smiling. Her hands begin to roam more freely and bravely across your shoulders, back, and down your arms. You can feel her breath on your neck.

Do what you are describing. Caress your partner's back and arms, and breathe on his neck and into his ears.

You watch in the steamy mirror as the maid leans over to roll down her stockings. She unties the ruffled white apron and lets the silky black of her dress separate and fall to the floor. You stare at her shapely body and smile when you see that, after all, she wasn't wearing any panties. You watch in the mirror, amazed, as she strolls confidently around to the front of the tub. She lowers herself into the water, and you see first her short pubic hair and then her full breasts disappear under the surface.

Stand up beside the bed and remove your clothing to reveal your naked body. Take your partner's penis in your hands, and lightly squeeze his testicles.

The maid glides closer to you, and you feel a pang of pleasure as she firmly takes hold of your cock underneath the water, then reaches below to squeeze your sensitive balls. Holding on to your shaft, she pulls you across the tub on your knees until you are directly in the path of a jet of water. She aims your cock straight into the gentle jet of warm, rushing water. Its swollen head feels as if hundreds of needles are gently piercing it with pleasure. It's almost too much.

Tell your partner to really imagine what it would feel like to have the jet of water on his penis. If you have one, he may want to try it out. Get back onto the bed and slide behind your partner. Press your breasts against his back, and reach around to stroke his penis. This should feel wonderful for you, so let him know.

The maid slides behind you and presses her wet breasts against your bare back. With one hand, she continues to aim the head of your cock into the softly surging water. With the other hand, she reaches down and begins to lightly run her fingers around your anus. She's on her knees behind you, moaning into your ear as she stimulates you in a way you've never felt before.

Whisper huskily into your partner's ear. Nibble at his earlobe while you speak, and push the tip of your tongue into his ear.

She whispers, "I have to let you in on a little secret. I noticed your wedding ring. Some of the other maids and I play a little game with some of the more attractive married male guests. Would you like to know how the game is played? First, we do our very best to make him come in the tub with the best hand job of his life. Most guys don't get past this point. If he does, we give him a blow job like no other. Any guy who can last through that without coming, I would fuck rather well. Are you game?"

The maid waits for your reaction, but you don't know how to react. You don't know if you should pretend to be insulted, when the truth is you feel incredibly turned on. You've never cheated on your wife and you never thought you would. Yet here you are, with a naughty French girl stroking your cock and pointing it into the jet of water. The warm, gentle pulses of the water feel like nothing else ever has. You know you could have an orgasm at any moment. But you want to keep playing the game. The maid does her best to make you come, stimulating both your cock and your ass at the same time. But you want to come in her, not in the water.

Begin to run your fingers and hands around your partner's genitals. Use some saliva as lubrication to give him a hand job as best you can from your sitting position behind him. You may not want to use lube, since you will soon be using your mouth. Don't make him come yet.

The maid grins in admiration and says, "No man has ever

made it through one of my hand jobs before. Your control is excellent. Why don't you sit on the edge of the tub? Your wife will never know ... it'll feel so good in my mouth that you won't believe it."

Tell your partner to sit on the edge of the bed. Kneel on the floor in front of him, and spread his legs open so you have access to his genitals.

This is when you need to make the temptation seem very real to your partner. Still kneeling between his legs, run your hands anxiously all over his body, including his genitals. Tell him you want him to really imagine how that temptation would feel. He's away from home, and a beautiful woman is offering to give him a blow job. And if he gets through that, she's offering even more.

"First you can have my mouth, then my pussy. Imagine the feeling against your shaft as my pussy slides against it. Imagine the feeling on the head as it breaks through and sinks into me. It'll feel warm and wet and tight. All you have to do is play the game. All you have to do is get through my blow job without coming. Then you can drive that incredible dick of yours as deep as you want into me. Just give in. You could be fucking me within minutes. Forget the guilt. It'll go away by morning. Surrender to the temptation—there's nothing like it. And nobody will ever know."

Stand up so your man can look at your naked body. Push against his chest so that he lies on his back on the bed, with his spread legs still hanging over the side.

You've never been so hard in your life. The maid stands up in front of you, water dripping off her breasts and small droplets hanging from her nipples. She pushes against your chest until you lie back. Your feet are dangling in the tub, but now you're lying on your back on the platform of the tub with your erection standing straight up, waiting for her mouth.

Make your partner wait for your touch. When you are ready, close your lips tightly, place the head of his penis against them, and push it through. Let your lips resist momentarily, then let his penis sink into your mouth as far as you can take it.

You squeeze your eyes shut, unable to fight what is happening. You feel her tight, warm lips against the head of your cock, and then you feel it plunge into her mouth. It goes the whole way in—she's deep-throating it.

Tell your partner to watch in the mirror.

Imagine the sight as you turn your head and look into the mirror. You can see yourself lying back with your feet in the tub, and this woman doing her very best to suck you off.

Perform oral sex on your man until he is very hard and you know he is close to coming. You're not going to make him wait much longer.

The maid tells you that you have passed the blow job. She can hardly believe your stamina, and she can't wait to fuck such a perfect cock.

Have your partner get up and stand beside the bed while you lie down on your back and continue the story. He can look down at your exposed body while you touch yourself.

The maid steps out of the tub and walks over to the bed. You stare at her naked ass as it moves away from you, and you notice a birthmark on it. It looks so different from your wife's ass, and all of a sudden you're struck by the reality of what is happening. Without any hesitation the maid pulls back the comforter all the way and lies flat on her back on the sheets. She spreads her legs wide and touches herself with her fingers. She tells you again that nobody will ever find out. She tells you it would be a shame to win the game but refuse the prize. And she reminds you how much she wants it. You get out of the tub and walk over to her.

Revive your partner's visual of where he is, and with whom, as he stands beside the bed, waiting for further instructions.

Imagine yourself standing naked beside the bed, looking down at this naked woman. She's lying flat, her legs wide open, waiting to feel you between them. You stare at her as she inserts a finger into her pussy. She pulls it out and you can see it's slick from her wetness. You've never been so desperate for another woman. You want to fuck her so hard. You want to show her just how good you really are. She whispers, "Just give in, it'll feel so good. It'll all be worth it."

You surrender to your desire, almost against your will. You can see yourself climb on top of her in the mirror, and again it's like watching a movie—it's so unbearably erotic. You feel the unfamiliar sheets against your skin. Everything is so different, especially the woman lying underneath you.

Have your man watch in the mirror as he positions himself on top of you, missionary style. Just as he is about to enter you, stop him. Climb up on your knees, and turn around.

The maid wants you to fuck her from behind. She tells you to fuck her as hard as you want. She likes it when a man grabs her hips and pulls her back forcefully onto him, especially a man with as much control as you. She's on her hands and knees in front of you, inviting you to enter her. Her ass is right in front of you, waiting. It's so round, and again you're struck by the re-

ality of what is happening when you see the birthmark on her ass. She looks different from your wife, and you wonder if she feels different too.

Because you have left a dim light on in your bedroom, your partner will be able to get a good look at you in this position. It will add a great touch to this fantasy if you have earlier applied a fake birthmark to your bum, or elsewhere if you already have one there. Men are visual, and it will be much easier for him to imagine a different body if yours looks a little different.

Let your partner enter you from behind. You want to get him as worked up as possible, so keep telling him to go harder and harder into you, providing that is something you enjoy. Remember that the bonus of leading him through the fantasy is that you get to pick and choose much of the action, so do what you're in the mood for.

You're fucking the French maid from behind as hard as you can . . . you're pulling back on her hips, entering her pussy with your cock. She's pushing back eagerly, longing for each and every thrust.

Be desperate and be loud as you reach orgasm. Tell him to stare at the birthmark and imagine he's penetrating another woman's body. Get your man going so fast and so hard that he can't help but come inside you. And tell him to watch in the mirror as he does.

You watch in the mirror as you fuck the maid from behind. Both of you are close to coming. A powerful orgasm washes over you and the come erupts out of you in waves. The maid loves the feel of your cock pulsing inside her, and she comes right after you do. You collapse onto the bed in exhaustion.

The maid climbs off the bed and smiles at you. She tells you that you're the best prize she's ever won. Now sated, she dresses herself and slips out of your room, blowing you a kiss as she leaves. She's on her way to brag to the other chambermaids. You're left alone to bask in the afterglow of your first-place finish.

AFTERWARD, tell your partner how good he made you feel and how much fun you had leading him through this fantasy. Compliment him on his exceptional technique, hardness, and of course his award-winning stamina. As always, share a laugh over the fantasy. Maybe place a mint on his pillow and tell him to come again soon. Or, present him with a FIRST PLACE ribbon. Lie your man on his tummy, and treat him to a really good back-scratch. And as he falls asleep beside you, remember that the smile on his face is for you, not for the score-keeping French maid.

SEXY SNIPPETS

1. *The maid watches you walk out of the shower, and hands you a towel. You catch a glimpse of the garter belt under her short black skirt.*

2. *She strokes your cock under the water, and the jets of water pulse against the throbbing head.*

3. *You're sitting on the edge of the tub, and she's sucking hard with her full lips . . . it's so hard not to come.*

4. *She's on her knees in front of you on the hotel's king-size bed. You're entering her hard from behind.*

14

THE CAMPING TRIP

HAVE YOU EVER slept outdoors? The open sky, the solid earth, and the fragrant, musical air constitute something of a return to a more primal state. That state, especially under the canopy of a night sky, can rouse feelings of raw sexuality that many people revel in. In this fantasy, your partner shares his sleeping bag with more than mosquitoes.

The particulars of this scene depend on how much camping gear you own. If you were planning on purchasing camping items this season, now might be an opportune time. At a minimum, this fantasy could benefit from a sleeping bag big enough for two. If you have the equipment and the inclination, you can incorporate everything from a tent to hot dogs and marshmallows. The open sky is the limit. As always, if you don't have the time, resources, or interest in physically setting the scene, you can mentally lead your man through this fantasy by simply whispering it into his ear.

If it's summertime and you have a private backyard, you can go all out and set up a tent and sleeping bag in it. Serve hot dogs or hamburgers on tin camping plates and eat under the stars. If it's winter or you don't own a lot of camping gear, you can simply lay out a sleeping bag on your living room floor. Roast hot dogs in your fireplace if you have one, or just serve them on plastic plates if you don't. Have fun!

Even if you have just laid out a sleeping bag on the living room floor and dimmed the lights, your partner will know you're ready to play. Wear cutoffs and a bandana, or whatever you would wear camping. A button-up shirt is ideal for this role-play, as you will see.

Serve him his fireside dinner, and for dessert fry up a couple of buttered cinnamon buns—they're the perfect camping sweet and are probably something you don't indulge in very often. Preparing foods you don't normally eat is a great way to de-accustom both of you to your usual routine. Food and sex are life's most generous pleasures, and a meal or snack is a wonderful way to work into or wrap up any sexual experience.

After dinner, snuggle up to your partner. Reminisce about a camping trip you took together, dream about one in the future, or ask him if he went on any memorable ones before you were a couple. To allow you to gently ease into a more sexually oriented conversation, say something like:

Have you ever thought about having sex when you were camping? What do you think it would be like in a tent, or zipped tightly into a sleeping bag like this one?

Set the scene and get into the camping mood.

Imagine yourself out camping with some guy friends. Most of them have brought their girlfriends, but you're single and there on your own. It's a warm, starry night and the evening breeze is on your face. You're all sitting around the fire, and the air is filled with the snapping and popping of firewood. Little embers float into the air and burn out.

Your friends are sitting with their girlfriends on their laps. You can see they're feeling them up a bit. Everyone has had a bit too much to drink and it's made everybody frisky, including you. You don't have a girl on your lap, and you wish you did.

One by one, each couple gets up and climbs into the privacy of their tent. You watch jealously as they disappear behind the nylon flaps. You watch to see their silhouettes inside. You can see the outline of one of the girls pulling her top over her head, and you become even more envious.

Take advantage of this initial erotic image by touching your partner's body in a sexual way. Without getting too close to him just yet, run your hands over his chest, arms, and legs.

You wish you were going to crawl into a nice cozy tent with a nice cozy body. You wish you were going to end this night by getting laid, like your buddies. Every once in a while you notice one of the tents shake just before you hear muffled giggles from inside. You know what's going on, and that awareness turns you on even more.

You try to distract yourself from the fact that there's no way for you to have that kind of release tonight. You're going to be sleeping in a tent with one of your buddies and his girlfriend, so you know there's no way you could even masturbate in safety. They're in the tent right now. The tent is shaking so you know they're having sex, and you can't go to bed until you're sure you won't interrupt them.

Tell your partner to really imagine himself there, sitting by the fire late at night, while couples are having sex just beyond the thin nylon walls of their tents. Ask him how aroused that would make him.

After a while your buddy comes out and has another beer. He winks at you and you know he got lucky. He comes over to you and tells you that one of his girlfriend's friends is going to be crashing in the tent too. You feel a glimmer of hope, but then he tells you that the girl has a boyfriend. He couldn't make it because he had to work this weekend. You remember seeing the girl. She was kind of plain, but hiding a good body. But you know there's no chance you're going to get off tonight, and you resign yourself to the fact that you'll have to suffer through it.

The alcohol has given you a warm, glowing feeling that has unfortunately seemed to center on your groin. You decide it's best to just put yourself out of your misery, so you get up and stumble over the loose earth and bulging tree roots toward the tent. You slip through the nylon opening. Your sleeping bag is already in there and you struggle to climb into it. Your buddy's girlfriend is still in the tent, fast asleep. She's sated. You close your eyes and do your best to ignore the beginnings of a hard-on.

Begin to concentrate your caresses on your partner's penis. He should still have his pants, pajama bottoms, or underwear on, so rub his penis through the fabric.

Continue with the story.

You're just about asleep when you hear someone crawl into the tent. It's your buddy. You watch out of the corner of your eye as he squeezes into the same sleeping bag as his girlfriend. She's still sleeping, and he nuzzles up to her. Within moments his breathing changes and you know he's asleep too. Again you're just about to fall asleep when you hear the tent flaps separate and another body crawls into the small tent. It's the girl.

She sits up on her knees and looks around the tent, searching for a place to crash. She makes eye contact with you and whispers, "Hey, I don't have a sleeping bag." She motions to her sleeping friend and says, "She said I could borrow hers, but obviously she forgot." The girl looks a little shy and uncertain, but then risks it and asks, "Do you think I could squeeze in with you? I don't take up much room."

Rub your partner's penis with more pressure, and squeeze his testicles through the fabric of his clothing.

You look up at her. She's shivering from the cold and unsteady from the alcohol. She smells like the campfire, smoky and slightly musty, and her hair is in a ponytail. You say, "Sure," and she makes her way over toward you.

You unzip your sleeping bag and she squirms in, legs first. You're immediately struck by the closeness of this girl you don't know, and by the feeling of her body struggling against the sleeping bag and against you. While you're not overly attracted to her, the friction of her body against yours involuntarily makes you think about sex again. You automatically start to imagine what her naked body would feel like squeezed in so tightly beside yours.

Now press your body boldly against your partner. If you have a sleeping bag, your work is easy. Climb in and squirm, twist, and push against him in any way that feels good. A strategic push against his groin won't hurt, either. If you don't have a sleeping bag, try wrapping yourselves tightly in the bedsheets. Necessity is the mother of invention.

She's crammed in the sleeping bag with you. You're trapped against her. There's no way to escape or maneuver your body to avoid contact, and you start to worry that you'll never fall asleep. You struggle to turn your body so that she won't feel your growing erection, but the effort itself causes her body and the restrictive sleeping bag to rub against you and make you harder.

Revive your partner's visualization while you stroke his chest and groin.

Imagine yourself squeezed into this little cocoon with this girl, both of your bodies pressed shamelessly against each other. In any other circumstance this closeness between strangers would be unacceptable, but necessity has given it a certain legitimacy. And the alcohol is definitely contributing to this relaxed sense of morals.

The girl fights with her fleece sweater and finally peels it off over her head. She tosses it out of the sleeping bag and it lands somewhere in the dark tent. She quickly pulls the sleeping bag up around her neck and says, "Brrrrr." You don't say anything. You just want to fall asleep and not give the alcohol a chance to let you make a fool of yourself. You fight the growing impulse to rub your dick against her body. She whispers something about your not getting the wrong idea, and then quickly— almost too quickly—nods off to sleep, semitranquilized by the alcohol in her blood.

You lie there, soaking in the sensation of this girl's body forced up against yours. She's lying on her back, breathing deeply. You lift the covers slightly and peer down into the sleeping bag. She's wearing a blue cotton button-up shirt, the first couple buttons of which have come undone. You can see the curves of her breasts, and that sight sends blood to your groin.

Have your partner peek down at your breasts. Make sure that you have discreetly unbuttoned your top enough for him to partly see them.

You decide to risk it. You reach down and cautiously undo another button. Then another. Soon her shirt is completely unbuttoned, and she hasn't stirred. As carefully as you can, you pull it open. She isn't wearing a bra. Before you know it you're staring at her completely exposed breasts.

Instruct your man to unbutton your shirt and expose your breasts as carefully as he can. Close your eyes, and pretend to be asleep. Pretend it's really happening—you're squeezed into a sleeping bag with this man, and he's looking at your breasts while you sleep. Allow yourself to become lost in the eroticism of the idea.

You can see the pinkness of her nipples even in the darkness of the tent. You reach down and very softly touch the tip of a nipple with your finger. It's hard. You reach down with your other hand and quietly unzip your jeans. You pull down your underwear far enough so that you can stroke your cock.

If he doesn't take the initiative himself, instruct your partner to touch your nipples with his fingertips. Then have him unzip his own pants and pull his clothes down just enough to free his penis. Tell him to close his eyes and picture what you are describing as he begins to touch you and himself.

You're stroking your cock and it feels really good. You carefully take one of the girl's hands and move it toward your groin. It touches the head of your cock, and you can't believe how good that feels. You gently move her hand up and down the shaft, doing your best to wrap her limp fingers around it.

Wrap your hand around your man's penis and stroke him gently.

You want nothing more than to get off. Your erection is growing harder by the second and soon you don't trust your own cock. It could go off without any warning. But you don't know how you're going to do it. If you come, there's going to be evidence in the morning... the girl might see it on her jeans or on the inside of the sleeping bag.

You suddenly notice that the girl is starting to stir. You freeze. If she wakes up to find her shirt and your jeans wide open, she'll freak out. You hold your breath and stare at her.

Pretend to be stirring, but not waking. Move your hand slowly and begin to caress your breasts, pinching your nipples. Your senses should be heightened, and this will feel wonderful.

She doesn't wake up, but her hand begins to move toward her chest; she is probably unconsciously sensing the exposure. A hammer of intense pleasure strikes between your legs, and you have to swallow an audible moan as you watch her hand begin to move over her own breasts. She drags her fingertips over the smooth flesh, caressing herself. She stops when she touches a nipple, and she begins to pinch and rub it. A soft sigh escapes her lips. She's dreaming.

Tell your partner to open his eyes, and let him watch you lie back and caress your own breasts and nipples.

Your eyes dart around the tent to see if your friend and his girlfriend have woken up, but they seem to be in a deep sleep. You're nervous about getting caught, but you're so worked up that the fear subsides. You keep watching this girl touch her breasts, and you begin to touch yourself more aggressively. You're going to have to come, and you're not worried about the mess anymore. You'll deal with that in the morning.

It's painfully erotic to watch this girl having a wet dream and fondling her own breasts. You're so turned on that you can't stop yourself as you bend your head down closer to her breasts and lightly flick your tongue over a nipple. She lets out another sigh, and you pause, waiting to make sure nobody else in the tent wakes up.

Pull your partner's head to your breasts, and have him lick and then suck your nipples while you continue to lead him through the story.

When you're certain the other couple is still asleep, you move your lips back to the girl's nipple and start sucking it. You can feel her respond. She rocks her hips against your hips and your cock throbs from the direct contact. She shows no signs of waking up. For a fleeting moment you wonder if she's actually awake and just letting you do this to her.

Push your body against your partner's groin to make him harder, and to enjoy the feeling of his hardness.

You decide to get everything you can out of this, so you reach down and quietly unzip her jeans. You slip your hand inside. You can feel her wetness has soaked through her panties. Again you feel a bolt of pounding pleasure in your already stiff cock. You peer down but it's too dark to get a good look at her panties or her pussy.

The girl's legs spread automatically to allow you entrance. Slowly, cautiously, you slip one finger underneath her panties, and in one motion you insert it into her pussy. Another sigh, and her legs spread even more. She moves her hips forward as her body instinctively moves to meet your penetrating finger.

Guide your man's hand to your pants or pajama bottoms and slip them underneath. Spread your legs wide and push one of his fingers inside you, underneath your panties. Show him how good it feels, and remind him at regular intervals to close his eyes and actively picture himself crammed in a sleeping bag in a dark tent, fondling this dreaming girl.

You wonder what would happen if you stuck your cock in her, instead of just your finger. You wonder if she would move to meet that hard flesh too, or if it would be too big and she would wake up. You decide to play it safe and just jerk off on her. You start to stroke yourself harder and more deliberately, eager to come. You can feel your orgasm rising, and you keep your eyes glued to her breasts. They're shaking from your rhythmic motion.

Have your partner begin to stroke himself. Let him do this for a while.

Your orgasm continues to build and build. You're very close to coming when suddenly you hear movement. You freeze. From inside your sleeping bag you peek out into the tent toward the other couple.

Hold his hand so he cannot stroke himself.

A stab of panic hits you as you realize your buddy's girlfriend is wide awake and staring at you. You wonder how long she's been watching and how much she's seen. At any moment you expect her to get up and make a scene, but she doesn't. Instead, she just stays where she is, watching. A mischievous smile comes over her face, as if to say, "Carry on." You can't believe it. You can see her arm moving underneath her sleeping bag and you realize she's touching herself.

An almost animalistic desire comes over you at the thought of your buddy's girlfriend watching you fondle her sleeping friend. She's the voyeur, but you're as turned on by it as she is. She moistens her lips and keeps watching you.

Lean in close to your man, and whisper sexily into his ear. Breathe into it as you speak, and nibble his earlobe. You want him to experience the mounting tension.

You decide that you've come too far and done too much to stop now, so you might as well give yourself some release and get off. You probably wouldn't be able to stop yourself at this point anyway. You'll deal with the consequences tomorrow. The chances are good that since your buddy's girlfriend is getting off watching you, she won't say a word about it in the morning. You can both blame what you're doing on the alcohol and forget about it.

Have your partner again begin to stroke himself. Keep your hand on his, and bring him close to orgasm.

You start to stroke your cock again, and almost immediately you can feel your orgasm continue to build. You're basking in the intensity of it when the girl beside you stops touching her breasts and begins to move. You've already had your momentum broken once, and you don't want to stop again. You keep stroking yourself even as she opens her eyes and looks at you.

You're past the point of caring. Even if she freaks out you'll have enough time to come on her, and that's all that matters to you now. You have to have relief. You can't wait to feel the come explode out of you and wrack your body with pleasure. The girl keeps moving and you keep stroking. She smiles and reaches below, pushing her panties down just a bit. She rolls onto her side, facing you. She takes your cock in her soft hands, and places it between her legs, against her wet pussy, with a sigh.

Take your man's penis in your hands and direct it between your legs, sighing to express your pleasure. Pull your panties down a little, but do not let him enter you. Instead, keep his shaft pressed against your vagina and squeeze with your legs.

You feel the warm wetness of the girl's pussy against your shaft. "I have a boyfriend," she whispers, "so don't put it in. Just keep it on the outside." She squeezes her legs tightly around your cock, and the pressure feels wonderful.

The restrictive tightness of the sleeping bag or sheets around your bodies will add to the excitement of the fantasy. The fact that you still have some clothes on will also add a sexy unfamiliarity to your lovemaking.

Continue to whisper in your partner's ear as you bring yourself to orgasm.

You and the girl move and rock against each other slowly. It feels exquisite to finally feel warm, moist pressure around your cock. And she loves the hard thickness between her legs. She rocks against you, squeezing her thighs together to stimulate her clit. She savors each sensation as she brings herself close to orgasm. You feel a shiver run over her skin and she moans in your ear. She's coming on you.

Come whenever you like. Then continue on to bring your partner to orgasm.

You've made the girl come so hard. You hear a gasp from the back of the tent and you know the girl who is watching has also come. Your aching cock throbs with mounting pleasure as it glides against the slippery lips of your bag-mate's pussy. You can feel the elastic of her panties rubbing against the underside of your shaft as you thrust between her legs, fucking her on the outside. You feel your orgasm swell, and a current of piercing pleasure surges through your body as you come.

Your thrusts slow and gradually your orgasm subsides. You and the girl lie back in sexual contentment. She whispers a sat-

isfied "Thank you" into your ear, and rolls onto her other side. The two of you lie spooned together in the sleeping bag. At last, you are able to drift off to sleep in the fresh, cool air.

AFTERWARD, tell your man how good he made you feel. Tell him how exciting it is to have his penis between your legs, and how good it feels. Tell him that if he invests in more camping equipment, you'll make it worth his while. If you're hungry, get up and make pancakes or hot dogs. And as the campfire burns out, remember that the smile on his face is for you, his wonderful woman, and not for the cuddly camper.

𝒮EXY 𝒮NIPPETS

1. *You're stroking yourself in the sleeping bag, staring at her hard nipples while she sleeps.*
2. *You can't stop yourself as you bend your head down closer and lightly flick your tongue over a nipple.*
3. *She tells you that you can't put it inside, that you just have to rub it on the outside.*
4. *You can feel the elastic of her panties rubbing against the underside of your shaft as you thrust between her legs.*
5. *You throw your head back in ecstasy, and catch a glimpse of the girl at the back of the small tent watching you and touching herself.*

15

MOVIE NIGHT

HUS FAR these fantasies have involved nameless, faceless women. Now it's time to put a face on the fantasy, and nowhere will you find a more beautiful face than in the movies. Most men have a favorite actress whom they feel is particularly stunning or sexy, and in this fantasy your partner is her leading man—in an X-rated love scene, of course.

This fantasy is called Movie Night because that's precisely what it should be. To be consistent with the theme, choose a weekend evening. Many couples rent movies at home almost every weekend, so this fantasy allows you to break out of the routine and make your regular movie night something special. To make your partner anticipate your evening in advance, slip a SPECIAL SCREENING TONIGHT ticket into his lunch box or pocket so that he can unexpectedly come across it during the day, and wonder what you have in store for him when he gets home. To prepare, visit the video store and rent a movie or two that stars your partner's favorite actress. For dinner, prepare only food that is served at the movies; hot dogs and nachos with cheese are great, since most men love these things anyway. Serve them on paper plates.

For snacks, prepare fresh-popped popcorn and have ready soda, licorice, chocolate bars, or whatever your partner usually buys at the movies. Put the popcorn in small paper lunch bags, and use lots of butter and popcorn seasoning. Arrange all the food and snacks on the coffee table, lower the lights in your living room, and cue the movie. If you have a television in your bedroom, you can prepare everything by the bed using nightstands or food trays for the snacks.

For extra effect, set up your own video camera next to where the action is going to take place. You don't even have to turn it on. Its mere presence will be enough to stimulate your imaginations and contribute to the eroticism of the encounter.

Finally, unplug the phone. We repeat: unplug the phone. That includes the cell phone. They'll call back, we promise.

When your partner comes home, tell him that instead of going out to the movies, you're staying in to the movies. Your efforts to make this movie night special will not be lost on him, and already this normally predictable night will be something fun and different. The few simple changes you've introduced into your routine will dress up any casual movie night.

Curl up on the couch or on your bed and watch, cuddled together, in the dark. Throughout the movie, shower your man with little kisses and affection, and ask him to put his arm around you—just like at the movies! When his favorite actress comes on the screen, innocently ask:

Isn't that the actress you think is so sexy? What's sexy about her?

Ask this in a playful and unthreatening way to show your partner that it's okay for him to answer honestly. If the movie is a sexy one, your work is easy. If not, you may have to steer him toward sexy thoughts. You can turn the conversation sexual by pondering aloud the logistics of a movie love scene.

I wonder what really goes on when they film love scenes in movies. Do you think the guys ever really get hard? I mean, if you were making out with her in a love scene, do you think you'd get hard even if lots of people were around?

If there is a sexy scene in the movie, you can talk about that one and have your partner imagine himself in it. If not, you can make one up. For example, you can set up the fantasy by saying something like:

Imagine that the cameras and workers are all around you, and you're sitting next to her on a bed. She lies down in a sultry way that says, "I want you, come take me." She's a very convincing actress, and in the scene she's doing her best to get your character to have sex with her. She's supposed to seduce you and make you unable to resist her.

Lean in a little closer to your partner, begin to caress his body more, and slide your body under him so you are in a sexually suggestive position that similarly says, "Come on, take me."

In the script she convinces you to take her clothes off.

Take your man's hands and guide them to your body. Show him that you want him to undress you while you continue to lead him through the fantasy.

While you're taking her clothes off and anticipating what she looks like naked, she reaches out and begins to undo your pants.

Now you can undress your partner completely.

I want you to imagine you're a famous actor and I'm that actress. Nobody knows, but you're attracted to her and you're really enjoying doing this nude love scene. You're worried the set crew will see your growing erection, and you're especially worried she's going to feel it.

By now both you and your partner should be naked.

She reaches up to you and pulls you down toward her own naked body. Instantly you feel the warmth of her unfamiliar form underneath you, and the softness of her smooth skin against yours. You lower your body on top of hers all the way.

She tells you she wants you so bad that she can't wait ... she opens her legs wide and begs you to take her right now. You're supposed to climb on top of her and move up and down, just mimicking sex. You're supposed to pretend that you're fucking her. You climb on top of her, between her legs, but your erection accidentally touches her. You stop for a split-second, but she doesn't miss a beat. She's a professional and she wants to make this scene as realistic as possible.

She reaches down and grabs your stiff cock. She guides it to her pussy, and with one hand on your back she pushes you to enter her. You're surprised to discover that she's already wet and that your cock sinks into her pussy easily.

Of course, you too should be following the script. Feign surprise when you feel your man's erection, and follow that by putting a hand on his back and encouraging him to enter you.

You're thrusting in and out of her, for real. The set is com-

*pletely silent, and you know the crew can't believe what they're
seeing. Only porn stars really have sex on film, and you can't
believe this popular, beautiful movie actress is having sex with
you in front of all the crew and with all the lights and cameras
around you. And she's either really enjoying it or she's giving
an award-winning performance. She's moaning and dripping
wet. She meets all your thrusts with equal force and desire.*

Imagine yourself being filmed like this while you have
sex, and remind your partner of the cameras recording his
thrusts.

*You can hear the hushed whispers of the crew and the hum-
ming of the cameras as you thrust into her waiting pussy.
Suddenly you feel a surge of moisture and you know you're
making her come hard. You look into her face—her mouth is
open and her back is arched—and you don't know if she's doing it for the cameras or because it feels so good. She asks you to
come inside her, and you realize that line isn't in the script.
That makes you push all the harder until you're ready to do
what she says.*

Meet your partner's thrusts with enthusiasm until he
comes. This fantasy is simple, short, and sweet, and so should
your lovemaking be. "Movie Night" is as much about jazzing
up your routine and spending a fun night together as it is
about having sex.

*The cameras stop rolling and the sexy star nibbles your neck.
She whispers, "You deserve to win Best Actor for that performance."*

AFTERWARD, tell your man how much you enjoyed co-
starring with him. Tell him that, whatever the studio is paying him, it's not enough. Let him know how good he made

you feel, and how much fun you had with him on your night in at the movies. And remember that the smile on his face is for you, not for Ms. Hollywood Hottie.

Sexy Snippets

1. *You're supposed to climb on top of her and move up and down, just mimicking sex.*
2. *She reaches down and grabs your stiff cock, guiding it into her pussy.*
3. *You can feel the surprised eyes of the crew on your back as you thrust yourself into her again and again.*
4. *Both of you know you're not supposed to be doing this, but it feels too good to stop.*
5. *You've had this woman a hundred times in your fantasies, but now you're fucking her for real.*

16

OUR FIRST DATE

*I*F YOU and your partner had sex on your first date, this fantasy will not work for you. Skip it. If you did not, you can bet your new boyfriend thought about you in a rather compromising way after he dropped you off. The chances are stellar that he went home, fantasized about the date ending differently, and masturbated while thinking about you. In fact, you may have done the same. In this fantasy, your partner gets the long lost opportunity to have sex with you on your first date. You are going to suspend the laws of Space and Time for his benefit.

If you and your partner do not already have a regular date night set aside for just the two of you—no kids, phones, or dogs—get one. Go all out. That means hip hair, good makeup, fashionable clothes, and delicious perfume. The works. It'll make you feel as good as you look. An added bonus is that your partner will likely respond in kind, and you'll get to see him at his best every now and then.

While you are out enjoying your date night and your man is gazing in admiration at the goddess he is with, ask him if he remembers the first time you went on a date together. Remind him what you were wearing, where you went, what you ate, and so forth. If you don't recall, no matter. Just fill in the blanks to make yourself look even better.

The goal is to make you and your partner relive the feelings of newness, passion, and sexual tension that grace the early stages of a romance. You want to summon the memory of that anxious and desperate drive to discover the other person in every way, as well as the lustfulness that accompanies new relationships. You want both of you to reexperience the physical ache you had for each other in the beginning. This fantasy will allow you to indulge in that ache, and to experience it in a way that you couldn't at the time.

In this fantasy, the real object of your partner's desire is only inches away, and he can have you now in a way he could only fantasize about then. In this fantasy you can return to a time when the two of you were strangers to each other, a time that is in the past but that should never be forgotten. It is part of your history and of who you are today. And your partner was really, really horny. We guarantee it.

Spend the evening reminiscing about the force of those feelings so that by the time you get home, your partner is ready to act on them. When you get home and are ready for bed, don't change into your pajamas. Instead, stall for time while you begin to lead him through this fantasy. Ultimately he will undress you as your erotic storytelling proceeds.

Tell your man how much you enjoy thinking about your

early days as a couple. Playfully reveal to him that you often had naughty thoughts about him after your dates, and ask him if he ever had them about you.

You can say something like:

After our first date, I distinctly remember having this warm, glowing feeling all over my body. It was definitely a sexual reaction to being out with you and from being attracted to you. Everything was so new. We were basically strangers, but I couldn't help wondering what you looked and felt like under your clothes.

You were so close, sitting right beside me, but we couldn't touch each other yet. I kept thinking about all the things we would do, or that I hoped we would do. I never thought such graphic things about other guys I went out with. They just dropped me off and that was the end of it. But it was different with you.

Make your partner feel like he was and still is special. Tell him you've never felt so sexually drawn to another man.

I remember lying in my bed and closing my eyes, picturing your face and your body in front of me. I remember imagining that I was peeling off your clothes, piece by piece. You probably weren't even home yet, and already I was in my bed, touching myself and thinking about you. I was dying to know what it would feel like to touch you—what your skin would feel like, how your lips would taste. I remember wondering what your arms would feel like wrapped around me, and how your weight would feel pressing down on top of me.

Your confession should make your partner feel comfortable enough to divulge his own secrets about the hours following that first date. If he reveals to you that he masturbated, ask him the details. After you have the particulars, you can act them out with him, or you can let him think about them while you have sex. You can also act out the things *you* imagined doing with him at that time.

Alternatively, you can proceed to lead your man through a fantasy version of what might have transpired that night.

You can try saying something like:

Imagine you're driving me home after our first date, and I ask you to come in for a drink. We hardly know each other. We've been sitting close all evening long, and many times your imagination ran away with you. You pictured yourself reaching out to touch my breasts, or leaning in to kiss my mouth. We've both endured strong sexual tension and attraction all night long, but now it's starting to weaken our resolve. Still, you're pretty sure you can control yourself, so you agree to come in for a while.

Make sure to sprinkle a few real details of that evening on top of your fantasy description. Seasoning any fantasy with actual facts or recollections will make it more accessible and realistic to both of you.

Begin to caress your partner's body and look into his eyes.

You walk into my apartment and I shut the door behind you. We've been out in public all night, surrounded by lots of people. This is the first time we've ever been alone together, and we're both acutely aware of the privacy we now have. The apartment is quiet and the silence adds to the sexual tension between us. We don't know each other that well, and we're kind of awkward together. I ask you if you want a drink or some coffee, and you accept.

I bring your drink and we sit on the couch in front of the television. I turn the TV on just to break the silence. There's some generic movie on and we stare blankly at it. This environment is new for us; conversation is a little strained. We're sitting very close and no one is around to see what we do. We're adults, so we can do whatever we want. We're just engaged in small talk, back and forth. Our conversation is uneasy.

Liberally add your own anecdotal comments about how attractive you found him. Describing your own feelings of mounting desire that night will increase his own. It will also turn you on by bringing back those feelings.

I can feel my cheeks are flushed. I'm thinking about all the things that could happen between us right now; and my body is responding. A couple times I trip on my words because of my distracted thinking.

Images flash across my mind. I see you leaning into me and kissing me passionately on my throat. I see you frantically pulling my blouse up and reaching underneath, feeling for my breasts. In my mind I can feel your palms pressing against my hard nipples. I see myself succumbing to you by sliding down onto my back on the couch, and waiting for your weight to pin me down.

Let your partner watch you touch yourself through your clothing while you are describing your feelings.

I shift my body on the couch so that I am facing you instead of the television. I like the sensation of being so close to you. I imagine myself sitting in front of you naked, my breasts exposed, anticipating your touch. That would feel so good. My breath and my pulse quicken at the image, and I'm sure you notice the change in my body.

You begin to hold my gaze longer now. Before, you'd only look at me for a moment, and then look away. It's hard to main-

tain eye contact with someone you barely know. We still are strangers, but now it's getting harder to pull our eyes away from each other.

I can feel my chest rise and fall. I'm becoming aware of the pattern of my breathing. I catch you looking at my breasts as they move up and down, and I can feel your eyes caressing them. I feel warmth between my legs and I know my panties are getting wet. My eyes are drawn involuntarily to your groin. I can see a bulge, and that fills me with nervous excitement.

Touch yourself with more urgency, and move your body in any way that feels—and looks—sexy.

You seem to experience the same sensations as me. You can feel my eyes touching your cock, and you imagine my tongue licking your shaft. Blood surges toward your groin and you feel the beginnings of an erection. Your cock stiffens and strains against the restriction of your pants.

Reach over and caress your partner's penis, either reaching into his pants or tracing your fingers over the bulge. Stroke his inner thighs and whisper throatily into his ear.

You don't want this to happen. You don't want me to think you just want to fuck me, so you get up to leave, hoping I won't notice your hard-on. You tell me you have to get home because you have to work early. Your voice shakes when you speak, and you find it difficult to stand up. Your legs seem weak.

I walk you to the door. There's a palpable tension, a strong pull between our bodies that makes it excruciating for us to separate. Every natural instinct and drive in our bodies is demanding that we come together. You're standing at the door, and we're saying good-night to each other.

Take a moment to review the big picture and bring it into sharp focus for your partner. Remind him that this is how your first date could have ended, and tell him to imagine how incredibly sexual and intense that would have been.

You lean in to give me a quick kiss on the cheek, but I turn my head and you kiss my lips instead. My forwardness makes your groin ache and you can't help but wonder what I'm thinking, and what I want. You decide to play it safe and begin to put your jacket on. You're just about to walk out the door. You turn to say one last good-night, but you stop in your tracks when you realize I'm unbuttoning my blouse.

You want your man to vividly remember how much he wanted you back then, and to reexperience seeing your exposed body for the first time. You want him to imagine how sexually raw and powerful it would have been had the two of you surrendered to your desires on that first date.

Again, since you have a pivotal role in this fantasy, you must describe your own thoughts and sexual urges as well as his. It was mutual sexual attraction—that is what fuels this fantasy, and that is what will turn both of you on. For most of us, the knowledge that we are desired by another person increases our own feelings of desire. Let your partner know how much you wanted him.

I don't want you to go and my body won't let you. It'll do whatever it takes to stop you from walking out that door. I have to feel your hands and skin on my body, I have to know what that would feel like. I know you share the same curiosity and I know you're feeling the same pull to stay. I unbutton my blouse, keeping my eyes locked on yours. You take your jacket back off and watch me.

Remove your blouse, but leave your bra on.

As you continue the story, have your partner undress you as you are describing him doing in the fantasy:

I stand in front of you in the doorway wearing my bra. You reach down and unfasten my pants (or skirt, or whatever you were wearing). *You pull them down and I step out of them. It's clear to both of us now that we are surrendering to our bodies. You remove my panties without saying a word. You see my pussy for the first time. You've been picturing it in your mind all night long.*

You reach behind me and unclip my bra. I feel my breasts slip free of it and now you see my breasts for the first time, too. Can you remember how it felt to see my pussy and my breasts that first time?

Ask your man to remove your bra. As he does, ask him to tell you how it felt to do that for the first time. Bring the memory and the sensations to the front of his mind. Tell him how exciting it was for you to expose yourself to him for the first time.

Still saying nothing, you stare at me, now standing completely naked before you. You know you have me. You know you can do anything. Your cock is rock hard, pushing against your pants.

Ask your partner if he could have resisted you if you had offered yourself to him like this on your first date. Hold back and give him a chance to seriously consider this. Just thinking back and imagining a different outcome to the evening should turn him on. Tell him some erotic details of what you did that night after your date. Tell him how you lay awake for hours, thinking of all the things the two of you could be doing together.

When you are ready, return to the fantasy.

I'm standing naked in front of you, offering myself, waiting to see what you'll do. You take my bra, place it between my legs like a sling, and then pull it back and forth against my pussy, rubbing my clit. I feel my pussy throb and pound from the fabric sliding over my clit as you rub me with my own bra.

If you want, ask your partner to stimulate you with your bra in this way. Continue with the story.

I arch my back in ecstasy. I lean back so that my body is pressed against the wall. You still haven't said a word, but you've decided that you're going to fuck me. You haven't even been inside my apartment before, but now here you are, ready to fuck me in it.

You strip quickly and furiously. Your cock is so hard and so big, and it's poking straight out from your body. I can't take my eyes off it.

Have your man remove his own clothes. Stand against the wall and stare at his penis with longing and admiration. Tell him it's perfect, and make him know that you can't wait to have it inside you. Tell him that you remember the first time you saw it, how gorgeous you thought it was, and how you wondered what it would feel like going inside you.

Continue with the fantasy.

You're not thinking about anything but fucking me as fast as you can. You were so polite and reserved all night on our date, but that's all gone now. All the pleasantries are gone. You wanted me all night, just like I wanted you. And now it's really happening.

As with most of these fantasies, there are any number of ways you can make your partner come; work your preference into the story.

If you and he are physically fit and compatible, you can have intercourse standing up, with your back against the wall. This "quickie" position screams naughty, gotta-have-it-now sex.

Say something like:

You push me back roughly against the wall and come at me. Your cock is digging into my stomach and I know any second it'll be in me, making me feel like nothing else can. You shove it in me and fuck me as hard as you can against the wall.

If you and your partner cannot comfortably have sex standing up, consider doing it with your body leaning over the bed or dresser, and him entering you from behind. This position is also fairly raunchy and lots of fun.

Say something like:

You grab me roughly by the wrist and pull me down the hall. You don't know where my bedroom is, but you find it and push me down face-first onto the bed (or dresser, whichever you prefer). You press my head down with one hand, and grab my ass with the other, moving it into position. You shove your cock in and fuck me as hard as you can.

Adopt whatever position you have chosen in the fantasy, and let your partner enter you.

My eyes are squeezed shut as your cock slides in and out of my pussy. I've never felt anything like it. It feels hard enough inside me that I think it could crack me open. I feel so full inside, and you're so swollen that you're taking up every inch of me. You still haven't said a word. You just keep slamming your big cock into my pussy from behind. You're ramming it into me and I can feel my orgasm building. I come so hard that the orgasm shakes my body.

Make a big production out of coming. Moan, scream, wriggle, and meet his thrusts with desperate, longing zeal. This will enhance your own orgasm, as well as your partner's.

You feel my juices slide down the shaft of your cock and over your balls. It makes you wilder, and you summon all your strength to pound me until you come.

Continue in this way until your man comes.

AFTERWARD, tell your partner there was no way in hell that really would've happened, but that it's fun to think about anyway! This fantasy gives you a wonderful opportunity to reminisce about your beginnings as a couple.

Tell your partner how wonderful he made you feel, and that you hope you made him feel good, too. Tell him you love your life together. Tell him he's the only man you've ever loved like this, and thank him for giving you such wonderful memories. Let him know your relationship is a priority in your life, far above everything else. And remember that the smile on his face is for you alone.

SEXY SNIPPETS

1. *I wanted you so badly. I tried to picture what you'd look like naked.*
2. *Can you remember how it felt to see my breasts and pussy that first time?*
3. *Imagine if we'd given in, if we'd fucked that first night, how intense that would've been.*
4. *I pictured you massaging my clit with my bra, pulling it back and forth between my legs.*
5. *I pictured myself lying face-down on the bed, and you ramming me from behind.*

17

THE MAIL-ORDER BRIDE

Part One

A S WE SAW in the previous fantasy, the combination of sexual tension and the natural awkwardness between strangers can be very arousing. In this two-part fantasy, your partner will find himself lying in bed next to a woman who is expected to satisfy him in every way—namely, his wife. The twist is that they have never laid eyes on each other before this day. Nonetheless, she is socially and legally compelled to be intimate, and your partner wants to enforce his rights!

In Part One, your partner will seduce his new and hesitant virgin wife until she is compliant enough that he can satisfy himself; however, he will leave her hanging and longing for her own release. In Part Two—which takes place the following night—he will bring her to such an overwhelming state of arousal that she is unable to resist anything he does to her body, including making her experience her first orgasm. Your partner will love the feeling of sexual power this fantasy exploits, as well as the idea of seducing and deflowering this inexperienced woman, despite her own initial reluctance. If you abandon yourself to your role, you also may love the feeling of sexual exploration and surrender this fantasy provides.

If you would like to act out parts of this love scene, strive to make your body appear somewhat different to your partner. As you did when you were the maid in the five-star hotel, you can add a birthmark to a part of your body. You can also apply a fake tattoo, as you did when you were your partner's amorous masseuse in the very first fantasy in this book. Because you are from a faraway land in this fantasy, you should choose a more exotic-looking tattoo, perhaps something patterned or Far Eastern. There are some lovely designs that will make your body your partner's temple.

As with many of these fantasies, you should also buy a new nightie. It should be something very conservative, such as an ankle-length, long-sleeved white cotton nightgown. Wear cotton panties. You are going to play the nervous, innocent virgin bride, so look the part. Present yourself as if the last thing you want to do is attract sexual attention, although that's exactly what you're going to get from your new husband. Wear a perfume that your partner won't recognize to further help him imagine you are someone else. Do whatever you can to make your body more easily seem like someone else's.

When both you and your man are tucked into bed together, fabricate something to introduce the topic of mail-order brides.

You can say something to the effect of:

I was on the Web today, and you know what I accidentally came across? Mail-order brides. Would you believe they actually advertise that stuff on the Internet now? It's like an online catalog, I guess. They had photos and descriptions of the women, along with their personality profiles and what they hoped to get out of a relationship, stuff like that.

Feign some playful curiosity.

What kind of man do you think would send away for a mail-order bride?

Discuss this with your man. It's a genuinely intriguing topic, and both of you will probably enjoy a conversation of this nature. The very idea of mail-order brides, and the forced, artificial intimacy the practice results in, naturally leads to sexual thoughts that you can take advantage of.

Now pose the inevitable question to your partner.

Do you think you would ever send away for one? I mean, can you picture yourself being at a time or place in your life where you would seriously consider it?

Your goal is to get your partner seriously thinking about this. This kind of self-reflection and study is almost voyeuristic, and he will probably enjoy it. You want him to really imagine himself at a point in his life where he might actually ponder a mail-order bride, even if only in a fantasy.

Imagine that you're single, you have a good job and lots of friends. But you're getting a bit older, and all your friends are married already. You feel like you're getting left behind. There are no prospects. All the women your age are already committed, and you can't find anyone you're interested in. Plus, you haven't been with a woman in a long, long time. What you want more than anything is to have a warm body beside you in bed. You fantasize about being able to just reach out in the night and touch a woman's smooth leg beside you. You fantasize about having, within arm's reach at all times, a woman to satisfy you sexually.

It's been so long since you've been with a woman that sex is always on your mind, and you're always longing for it. You've thought about prostitutes, but you want something more permanent. You want a woman of your own, a woman who can fulfill all your sexual needs and desires. She'll do whatever it takes to keep you completely satisfied.

You can now set the scene for the fantasy.

Picture yourself at the office one day, working on the computer. An e-mail comes in, one of those junk e-mails, and you go to delete it. Just before you hit Delete, an image fills the screen that grabs your attention. It's an online catalog for mail-order brides.

There are rows of full-length photographs of the women. They're of all nationalities. All you have to do is select one, and she'll be at your door in a matter of days. And after that, she'll be in your bed. It's been forever since you've lain next to a woman in bed, and you can't help but think that in just a few days you could have one beside you. Any one you want.

Playfully ask your man which nationality he thinks would interest him or draw his attention. After he has told you, quickly construct a visual of this woman in your head and describe every detail about her to him. Be sure to include hair and eye color, body shape, the size of her breasts, and any distinguishing features like birthmarks or tattoos—particularly any that you have already placed on your own body. Remember that your task is to provide your partner with the details, so be thorough and give his mind's eye a clear picture of this woman.

You decide to go through with it. You go through the motion's quickly without thinking about it, in case you'd talk yourself out of it. You select a woman, fill out the necessary forms and documents, submit them, and wait.

Only days later you get the call. It's the agency, and they tell you to pick up your bride at the airport tonight. You feel a stab of panic. You start to wonder what you were thinking, how you could have been so stupid. You wonder what you got yourself into, and how you're going to get yourself out of it. But then your thoughts turn to what this means for you. It means that tonight, this very night, only hours away, you're going to have a soft, warm woman lying beside you in your own bed.

You think about it all day long. She's come all this way and made this drastic change to her life in order to come to this country. But all you care about right now is that she's going to have to sleep in your bed tonight, beside you. And she'll know what's expected of a wife.

Do your best to make sure your partner is really imagining himself in this situation. You want him to feel the tense uncertainty, the fear of the unknown, and the thrill of it. You want him to picture himself driving to the airport in his car, picking her up, and bringing her home, to his own house, where she is expected to be his wife in every way. He must have a strong visual sense of himself in this situation and with this woman, in order for the fantasy to be at its most effective.

Imagine yourself driving to the airport. It's late already, and your nerves are raw from the hesitation and the excitement you feel. On one hand you wish you had never gone through with it, that you could make it all disappear. On the other hand you won't be able to get her in the car and in your bed fast enough.

Snuggle in close to your partner, trace his skin with your fingers, and let him become lost in the fantasy world. You too should be losing yourself in the story. Imagine that you're this awestruck, uncertain young woman, about to meet her new husband for the first time.

You stand at the meeting point in the airport and watch as the passengers file past you. Finally you spot her. She's dressed neatly in a simple skirt and white blouse. Her nipples are hard from the cool air of the airport terminal, and you can see them poking through her blouse. She's more attractive than her photo made her seem, and you feel a swell of arousal as you realize you'll be fucking her within hours. It's your wedding night, after all.

You approach her and she smiles timidly. She seems very sweet, very friendly. You like her. Her English is poor, very broken, and you can barely understand a thing she says. She doesn't understand you either, but you tell her she'll learn, not to worry. You pick up her bags and she follows behind you, out of the airport and into your car.

You get into the car together and drive away from the airport. You know she's uneasy from being so close to you in a confined space. She's alone in a car with a stranger, in a strange country, and you smile to reassure her. Her musky perfume fills the interior of the car as she stares straight ahead out the windshield.

You pull up to your house and carry her bags in. She's behind you, and when she steps into your house, she's in awe of what she sees. Obviously she's been very poor and has had nothing;

she's amazed by everything you have. She walks through the house, exploring. She looks in the fridge and can't seem to believe all the food you have at hand. She takes out some leftovers and looks at you for permission. You grin and nod. You want her to have lots of energy for tonight.

Recall that you are telling your partner these small details to make the situation seem real to him. The slow build will increase the level of his arousal as he anxiously awaits details of growing intimacy between himself and his bride.

As you tell the story, caress your partner, perhaps stroking the nape of his neck or tracing his lips with your fingers. You're telling a tall tale, so take time. Maybe treat him to a full-body massage as you speak—start with his scalp, move to his shoulders and back, then to his arms and legs. Don't forget his hands and feet.

She wanders into the living room and stares at the television. She doesn't even seem to know what some of the electronics are; she looks baffled. You follow closely behind her, watching her explore her new surroundings. Your chest occasionally brushes against her back and you can feel her ass briefly touch your groin. You really want to go to bed soon.

Finally, it's time to show her your bedroom. You both stand in the doorway and peer inside. There's an awkward silence as she stares at the bed. You're standing very close to her, and she turns to face you. You lock eyes for a brief moment, then she shyly looks away. You have an urge to throw her onto the bed and take her, but she looks so nervous and frail that you stop yourself. You can wait a few more minutes, until the time is right.

She disappears into the bathroom with her bags to get ready for bed. After only a moment she reemerges and, through a combination of hand gestures and foreign words, indicates that she doesn't know how to use the faucets. You lead her back into the bathroom, lean over the side of the tub, and demonstrate how the controls work. She offers a shy smile of gratitude, and you leave her. You hear the water running behind the closed door, and you hear it lapping around her body as she climbs into the full tub. You can picture her soaping up her soft skin, moving the slippery bar of soap over her breasts and between her legs. You like the idea that she wants to be clean for you.

You crawl into bed wearing only your underwear and stare at the darkened doorway, waiting for her to walk through it. She's been gone a long time and you know she's stalling because she's scared. You feel your cock twinge under the sheets. Her hesitancy and uncertainty make you want her even more. She looks so wide-eyed and innocent. A thought pops into your mind—could she be a virgin? The agency claimed she was, but you didn't actually believe them. You aren't that naïve. But just maybe...

It is now time for the reluctance element of the fantasy, and it is up to you how far you want to take it. If you oppose the idea of reluctance entirely, even in a fantasy, concentrate on the awkward unfamiliarity between the characters, and exploit that. You can present the mail-order bride as being highly attracted to her new husband and anxious to perform her wifely duties. Perhaps she is still a virgin, but cannot wait to try all the things she has heard about. Or perhaps she is very "worldly" in her sexual technique, and does things her new husband has never experienced.

Continue with the fantasy as you gently brush your partner's skin with your fingertips. Drag them lightly over every inch of his body, awakening and arousing his senses. This is a great way to follow the full-body massage.

You look up to see her standing motionless in the doorway to your bedroom. She's wearing a long white nightgown, and she has deliberately concealed from you as much of her body as she could. You're filled with lust for her, but you manage to produce a comforting smile. You pull back the covers and motion for her to come in.

She whispers something to you in her own language, and the foreignness of her voice entices you. She's seeking reassurance. You wonder if she's asking you for time. Maybe she doesn't want to rush it, she doesn't want you to take her on your first night together. But you just want to get her in your bed and do your best to convince her otherwise. Especially if she really is a virgin.

She lingers in the doorway and then, with faltering steps, walks toward the bed. You shift so she doesn't see your erection raising the covers. You don't want to scare her away. She eyes the empty spot in the bed beside you uneasily, and then bravely slips under the covers in one quick, decisive motion.

Stroke your partner's body with more pressure and urgency now, to ramp up his arousal. Both of you will be turned on by the ideas and images from your erotic storytelling.

She lies beside you frigidly for a second, and then flips over so that her back is to you. She wants you to ignore her and just go to sleep. You give her a moment, and then place the palm of your hand against the small of her back. Her body jumps at your unexpected touch. It's intoxicating to have this vulnerable, hesitant, beautiful woman lying beside you. You can tell that she's reluctant, but that some part of her is drawn to your touch.

If you're acting this part of the fantasy out, face away from your partner and let him touch your back in the manner described. Adopt an innocent disposition and, when he touches you, act as though you are frightened, but exhilarated.

Continue to lead your partner through the fantasy.

You start caressing her back with more determined and urgent strokes. You squeeze and hold her arm, using it to roll her over onto her back. She stares at the ceiling. She was expecting you to leave her alone, but now the reality of her situation is sinking in. She glances at you with concerned eyes, but you won't give up yet. You want her so much, and you know she wants you. She just needs to go slowly.

She whispers hoarsely in broken English something to the effect that she does not know anything about men. A charge of energy hits your unyielding erection and your cock feels as hard as concrete. You look at it and you're surprised at how big it seems, even to you. It's going to intimidate her. Now that you know she's a virgin, your body involuntarily moves toward hers in response to that irresistible knowledge. Not only are you going to fuck her, but you're going to be her first. You're going to be able to watch how she responds to every new sensation flowing through her body.

You've had enough of being patient. Now you're going to show her what's going to happen tonight. You have no intention of taking her forcibly. You want to seduce her. You want to make her experience new feelings that she won't be able to resist. You're going to have her, and she's going to want it. She's going to want you every bit as much as you want her.

Many men like the idea of deflowering a virgin, and if your partner is one of them he will love this fantasy. Similarly, it can be great fun for you to pretend that you are experiencing sexual feelings for the first time. Think back to what it was like.

You begin to rub her legs, moving up slowly toward her soft thighs. Her skin is warm and very smooth. You reach under the light fabric of her nightgown and caress her thighs. You move your hands up further, and feel her cotton panties. She lies motionless under your touch, reluctant and uncertain.

You spread her legs slightly open, and with your fingertips you touch the fabric of her panties. She draws in her breath and bites her lip. The newness of that sensation is shocking to her and she freezes for a moment. You place a soft kiss on her lips to reassure her, and she opens her legs wider. She wants more, despite herself.

Move your partner's hand under your nightgown and ask him to stroke and kiss you the same way.

You move your hand up further beneath her nightgown, over her smooth stomach. Finally your hand reaches the soft mounds of her breasts. You glide your hand over her breasts, rubbing your palm over each of her nipples and tweaking them with your fingers. Her breathing becomes shallow and she closes her eyes. You watch, captivated, as these first feelings of sexual arousal wash over her.

You sit up and pull at her nightgown, indicating that you want her to remove it. She clutches it to her breast, but you pull harder. She takes a deep breath, closes her eyes, and squirms out of it, still under the covers. She's naked under the covers, wearing only her panties, and lying just beside you. You reach out to feel her naked, smooth skin. She pulls away at your touch, nervous about her own exposed condition, but you move closer and keep touching her. Before long, she's turning her body toward you, just slightly.

Ask your man to take off your nightgown, but feign reluctance as he does.

You tug at the covers, but she holds onto them tightly. You pull them and she finally lets them slip away to reveal her naked body. Her breasts are full, and with instinctive modesty she brings her arms up to try and cover herself.

Have your partner pull the covers off of you in this way, again as you feign resistance. Clutch the covers and give him a bit of a fight!

She still won't look at you. She just keeps staring at the ceiling, as if she's pretending she's somewhere else. You imagine that she's wondering what is going to happen. You get up on your knees, and spread her legs open wide. You kneel between her open legs and slowly draw your eyes over every inch of her nakedness. She's perfect.

Have your partner get into this position, and have him continue to do what you are describing in the fantasy.

You're aroused by her body but you're even more aroused by her uncertainty. You place your hands on her and she tightens up. You begin to glide your hands over her legs, thighs, and arms. You want to relax her, get her into it. Then you begin to move toward her most private areas, the places you know she's wondering if you'll dare to touch.

You grasp her thighs, high up, and knead them in your hands. Her fingers clutch the bedsheets and her breathing becomes even more shallow and rapid. You apply more pressure and move your hands over her panties, touching her pussy underneath. She squeezes her eyelids closed tightly, trying to keep control of herself. The feelings are so strong, so unexpected. She can't believe a man is touching her like this.

Draw your breath in sharply when your man touches you

between your legs. Enjoy the idea of being touched there for the first time, and let him see that, in spite of his new wife's anxiety, she's becoming aroused.

You know it's the first time she's ever had hands on her pussy. You wonder if it feels good to her or if she's still too nervous. But something in the way she's holding her body makes you aware that she's curious.

You move your hands over her stomach and up toward her breasts. You cup a breast in each hand and massage it. Her body trembles. You take both her nipples between your fingers and again squeeze them hard. A sharp gasp escapes her lips and a shudder rocks her body. You can't tell which of you is surprised more by it. You can see her blink her eyes in amazement at the charge she just felt jolt through her body. You smile at her but still she doesn't look at you. You're extremely turned on by the fact you're giving her these feelings for the first time.

You slide your hand down between her legs and, without giving her any warning, slide a finger underneath the crotch of her panties to finally feel her soft pussy. It's wet, and your cock throbs as you realize she's getting aroused even in the midst of her uncertainty. You caress her pussy until you find her clit. It's swollen and slippery. She's getting wetter by the moment under your exploring touch, and her body is starting to move in surrender to her mounting feelings.

You should be wearing only panties and letting your partner explore you between your legs. Keep your panties on for the duration of Part One of this fantasy. When your partner ultimately penetrates you, move them aside to allow his penis entry.

You gently slip a pinkie finger through the pink lips of her mound. It's very tight. She bears down and tenses her body. She draws a sharp breath between clenched teeth, and you know she's never felt this before. Her pussy is so tight, you can't imagine how good it'll feel when you finally ease your cock into it. You gently push your little finger in and pull it out again and again, until it starts to emerge moist and shiny, and you know she's beginning to like it.

You try your middle finger next, and she arches her back in response, letting out a guttural moan. You look up at her face. She's biting her bottom lip. She still won't look at you, but she's not resisting, either. Your finger is getting wetter and wetter, and her hips are beginning to rock ever so slightly to meet your thrusting finger.

Guide your partner's hand between your legs and urge him to put a finger inside you.

You finger-fuck her for a while, pushing your finger deep inside her pussy and then pulling it out. It's slicker and wetter every time you withdraw it. She's embarrassed by her own arousal and doesn't want to reveal her excitement. You know she's still unsure, and her hesitation and reservation make your cock pound with agonizing pleasure. Your hips begin to rock back and forth, involuntarily mimicking the thrusting of penetration and withdrawal.

You grab a pillow and frantically push it under her ass so her pussy is higher up and more accessible to you. She braces herself, but doesn't try to move away. She knows what's coming but has no idea what it will feel like. You can't wait to show her. You're glad you'll be the first to show her.

Have your partner put a pillow under you in a similar way.

Pushing her panties aside, you lean over her and place the head of your cock at the opening of her sweet pussy. You try to push it in, but there's resistance. She's tight, but finally the head of your cock breaks through. It pulses from the pressure of her virgin pussy surrounding and squeezing it. She throws her head back and grabs at the bedsheets in pain and pleasure. You steady yourself and push again, harder this time.

Your cock plunges all the way into her pussy and you bury it as deep as you can inside her. She moans, and through your pounding pleasure you look at her face. She's blinking widely, stunned by what is happening between her legs and what it feels like.

When your partner enters you, play the anxious virgin and moan in shock at the unexpected pleasure.

You're just as turned on by watching her as you are by fucking her. It's her first time being fucked by a man and she's starting to like it. Ecstasy is starting to replace the pain. A flood of new feelings is washing over her untouched body, and you're the cause. You love watching it and knowing you're doing it to her. You're showing her how incredible sex is, and it's mind-blowing to watch.

Refresh your partner's visualization by having him look down to watch his penis entering and withdrawing from your body, underneath your panties.

Imagine yourself fucking this woman that you've only known for a few hours. She's lying in your bed and you're on top of her body, pushing your cock deep into her pussy. It's so tightly wrapped around your shaft that every time it plunges into her you feel like you could explode inside her. She gasps and throws her head back each time you sink into her. It's like she forgets what it feels like when you pull it out, but then remembers again when you push it back in.

She's never been with a man before, but you're changing all that right now. Your cock is the first one that's ever been in that tight little box. She's never known that sense of fullness and pressure in her body before, never experienced the weight of a man's body pushing down on hers. She's never before heard a man's heavy breathing and grunting in her ear while he drives his dick into her. She loves it. You look down and watch as your thickness disappears behind her panties, deep into her pussy. You're inside; but you haven't even seen her completely naked yet. It's captivating to watch your cock invade her panties. You were going to take them off, but there's no point now.

Let your man know that you want him to come—at his leisure, of course. Use the power of suggestion, describing to him how powerfully intense his orgasm will feel to both him and to the woman. This will make him anticipate his orgasm, and will increase its pleasure and intensity.

You feel your orgasm building. You know you've reached the point of no return and you feel the ache build in your balls. Come blasts out of you in wave after exquisite wave, arching your back and propelling your cock into her even harder. You're paralyzed by your orgasm and helpless to do anything until it subsides. You look down and see her panties become instantly soaked, drenched by both her own juices and your come. Her eyes are wide with pleasure and surprise as she feels your hotness gush into her.

If you can, wait until tomorrow night to come yourself. The anticipation and delay will make the experience of Part Two more intense for both of you. You can end Part One and simultaneously foreshadow Part Two by saying something like:

She wraps her legs around your body, wanting to satisfy herself. She wants to come, but you don't want her to. You want her to think about you all night and all day tomorrow. You want her to yearn for you before you take her again. Tomorrow night you'll give her what she needs in order to have her first orgasm.

(You should finish this scene while your partner is still inside you, enjoying the lingering effects of his orgasm.)

And so ends Part One!

AFTERWARD, tell your man what an irresistible seducer he is. Tell him how good his hands felt moving over your body, and how turned on you were by feeling and watching him penetrate you under your panties. Tell him how no woman in the world would be able to resist his sexual skill and technique for very long, and how lucky you are that you have it all to yourself. Stroke his ego and his penis. And remember that the smile on his face as he dreams the night away is for you, his adoring woman, and not for the mail-order bride.

SEXY SNIPPETS

1. *She's prettier than you expected, and the cold air of the airport is making her nipples hard.*
2. *You can hear the water lapping over her body as she steps into the full tub.*
3. *She's lying with her back to you, but you slip your hand underneath her nightie to feel her smooth, bare skin.*
4. *She lies frigidly, but under your touch her clit becomes smooth and slippery, as it swells from her growing arousal.*
5. *You look down and watch as your thickness disappears behind her panties, deep into her pussy.*

18

THE MAIL-ORDER BRIDE

Part Two

*P*ART TWO of this fantasy picks up where Part One leaves off. That is, with your partner's newly deflowered bride yearning for her first orgasm. Last night your partner took away her virginity and satisfied himself. Tonight, he will again satisfy himself—but now he will be a gentleman about it, and return the favor for his new bride. Tonight he will bring her to a level of arousal that will make her succumb to every one of his sexual advances. In this fantasy, chivalry is not dead, it has only been delayed. Lucky you!

You can begin Part Two of this fantasy by reminding your partner of Part One; review as much of it as necessary to arouse him.

After you have refreshed his memory, assume the position and lie next to your partner in your nightgown. Remember that you are the anxious bride, yearning for your first orgasm.

You can't wait for your new partner to reach over and again begin to do what he did last night. (If you yourself practiced delayed gratification and didn't reach orgasm last night, you should indeed be deliciously anticipating your partner's touch.)

Say something like:

Your new bride remembers very well what it felt like to have the weight of your body on top of her, and your powerful cock filling her tight little box with your juices. She wants to feel that again. She wants to feel that hard fullness in her pussy and the force of those thrusts against her body. She's still too shy to initiate anything, so she lies quiet and still next to you, anticipating your advances.

Lie next to your partner in anticipation. You long to feel his hands on you. Dare to reach out and touch his body. Make him know how badly you want him.

You don't have the willpower to make her wait very long, since you want to come again. Your orgasm last night was painfully strong. It wracked your body but left you wanting more, and you haven't been able to stop thinking about it all day. You pull her nightgown off over her head, and she offers only token resistance. Her breasts are full and waiting for your touch. She doesn't make any modest attempts to cover them tonight. She wants you to touch them.

Anxiously assist your partner in removing your nightgown to reveal your naked body.

You notice that she's already removed her panties. You stare shamelessly at her pussy. You couldn't see it last night, but now it's right in front of you, waiting. The hair is soft, in a natural downy triangle. You can picture her lying in the tub, cleaning herself, wanting to make it perfect for you—perfect for you to fuck. You brush the back of your hand over the soft hair and she gyrates her hips. She's clearly torn between putting on a show of modesty and just allowing your hands to explore her body and stimulate her.

Have your man perform what you are describing. Enjoy the feelings, and let your enjoyment show.

You lean over and flick your tongue over her nipples, and she arches her back. You see a faint smile on her lips for the first time, but she's still too nervous and too modest to surrender completely. That's okay. You know that by the end of the evening she'll surrender everything to you, and in any way that you want it. You know you did the right thing by making her wait until tonight. You have her exactly where you want her. And there's nowhere else she'd rather be.

You want this night to be something different. Not only do you want to bring her to orgasm, you want to overwhelm her with sensation. You want to bring her to a shaking, desperate peak; you want her to long for you and open up for you. Only you can bring her to orgasm. You're the only man in the world that can lead her body to that pleasure.

Tonight, you want to make her do all kinds of dirty things. You want to strip her of all her innocence and make her realize the power of sexual desire. You want to get her to the point where she'll do anything you ask, willingly and anxiously. She's so naïve, she has no idea of the power she could have over you. She has no idea of the things her body can do or feel, and you want to help her discover that sensuality.

If you are acting this part of the fantasy out, you will need to have ready the nipple clamps and vibrator you purchased for the sex-shop fantasy. Pull them out from under the pillow and continue to have your partner perform on your body what you are describing in the fantasy. If you're just whispering this fantasy in his ear, be very descriptive, to allow him to visualize the scene adequately.

You reach under your pillow where you have some things waiting for her. You place a pair of nipple clamps and a vibrator beside her on the bed. She has obviously never seen either of these things before, and she looks curiously at them. She's wondering what you're going to do, and you love the uncertainty and inquisitiveness in her eyes.

You place the first clamp on her nipple and she draws in a quick, loud breath. Her body begins to shake again from the newness of this kind of pleasure. She's completely caught off guard by her own feelings and seems to struggle with how to react to them. Should she resist them or should she give in and give herself to you? She wasn't expecting anything like this, you can tell. She was just expecting you to climb on top of her and fuck her again. She doesn't know what to do, or even if this is normal. Still, she's inclined to give you the benefit of the doubt.

You place the other clamp on her other nipple and stare down at her. Her body begins to move and squirm in ecstasy beneath you. Her legs are wide open and you're filled with intense desire as you stare down at her naked body with the nipple clamps pinching her hard buds. Her breathing is heavy and loud, and her breasts are heaving up and down.

Show your man that you want him to use the vibrator on you.

You deliberately want to overstimulate her, so you place the vibrator on her clit. She arches her back so high with pleasure that you have to press her body down and hold her still with your hand.

You should now have the nipple clamps on, and your partner should be touching your clitoris with the vibrator. Again,
be sure to act as vulnerable but lustful as you can. This is a
great fantasy and you want to get the most out of it.

*You turn the vibrator on "slow" and her body twists and
turns under you. You hold her as still as you can with one hand,
while your other hand continues to stimulate her. You explore
the folds of her pussy with the tip of the vibrator. You keep teasing her clit with the vibrator until you know she is ready to
come. You can hear her voice change and you can see her hips
moving rhythmically and desperately. But you don't want her
to come yet. You want her orgasm to build and build until she
explodes, so you pull the vibrator away from her.*

*She protests and pushes her hips toward you, begging you for
more. You take her hand and place the vibrator in it. You move
her hand toward her own pussy and indicate that you want her
to put it in herself. You can tell by the look on her face that she
is unsure about doing this. You suspect she's never masturbated
before and might not know what to do.*

*You push her hand into her pussy with more force, and she
gives in. She pokes the tip of the vibrator into her pussy, and you
reach down and turn the vibration up. She responds instantly,
and eases its shaft deep into her body.*

You should now be masturbating yourself with the vibrator. This will turn your partner on and allow you to stimulate
yourself in precisely the way you like. Make sure your partner is watching carefully, since you can use this as an opportunity to show him exactly what feels good for you.

*You sit back and stare down at her. The back of her head is
digging into the pillow in rapture and the nipple clamps are
shaking back and forth from the motion of her moving body.*

She is spreading her legs as open as she can, and she's fucking herself shamelessly with the vibrator. She's surrendered completely, and now she wants to feel the orgasm come over her.

The veins in your cock are pulsing hard with blood, and you're so turned on that you could come without warning at any moment. You position yourself between her legs, close to her pussy, and you're just about to take the vibrator out of her hand and penetrate her when you change your mind.

Instead, you reposition yourself so that you are straddling her torso, your legs on either side of her desperately writhing body. You reach behind yourself and take the vibrator out of her hands. Still reaching behind yourself, you wipe her palms against her pussy to get them wet. After they're wet, you direct her hands to your cock and wrap her fingers around it. She's so wet that she can use her own juices as lubrication while she strokes your cock.

Have your partner straddle your body. Wrap your hands around his penis, and begin stroking it. Just in case your own juices are not flowing with enthusiastic abundance, have some lubrication under your pillow. And don't get the bargain brand. The good stuff feels infinitely better.

You show her how you want her to squeeze your shaft with long, fast, hard strokes. She's never done this before, but she does it almost perfectly. She's squeezing so tightly that you know you're going to burst at any second. You reach around behind yourself again and push the vibrator inside her pussy. You fuck her with the vibrator as she squeezes and strokes your cock, coaxing you to orgasm. You look down at her, and she's loving it.

Your man should be straddling your body and using the vibrator on you. Show or tell him what feels good. You should be giving him a hand job, applying as much pressure as he can take to his penis. Have him also show you exactly what feels good to him, since you're just an uneducated virgin who wants to learn how to please her man. Be ready for him to ejaculate on you—aim his penis where he wants to come, or where you want him to come. The idea and the image of a man coming on a woman's body is arousing to many couples. If this is pleasurable to you, include it in the fantasy.

Although your partner will be very turned on already, be sure to reinvigorate his visualization at regular intervals. He will at times get lost in his own arousal, and you should occasionally lead him back into the particulars of the fantasy; specifically, where he is, with whom, and what he is doing. Give him the big picture. If your man can hear your voice describing the scene at the same time that he is experiencing the corresponding sensations, you will have mastered the art of erotic storytelling. You will strengthen both the force of the fantasy itself, and the intensity of your mutual arousal.

Imagine yourself on your knees, straddling this woman's body. She's squeezing your cock as hard as she can. It's close to her face and you have an image of come shooting out all over it. You're pushing a vibrator into her pussy. You only met her yesterday, and only yesterday you took her virginity. She was so pure, but now she's doing things she never even knew were possible. She's succumbed to your sexual knowledge and desires. She's given herself over to her pleasure and you hardly know each other.

You're high above her, looking down as she strokes your swollen, pulsing rod. You're so worked up that full, thick veins are clearly visible along your shaft. This woman's strokes feel inexperienced, but her desperation compensates for her lack of skill. Your orgasm is building, and the more it builds the harder you push the vibrator into her. She lets out a moan and you feel a rush of wetness run over the vibrator and your hand. She came. She's under your body as she comes, unable to escape the flood coming over her or the weight of your body pressing her against the bed. She can only wait for the orgasm to pass and release its hold on her.

Have your partner use the vibrator in any way that feels good and will bring you to orgasm. Take your time. You can bask in the view of his body above you, and at the same time delight in the sensations from the vibrator.

Her coming makes you come, and you feel your orgasm reach a peak as her hands continue to stroke and squeeze your cock. Any second you'll see the come blast out of you and onto her waiting body, covering her smooth bare skin with jism. Suddenly your cock erupts and come lands in waves on her body. Some lands on her lips and she laps it up, eager to taste her man.

Continue talking like this until your partner comes on you.

As your orgasm subsides and your other senses return, you look down at your new bride. She is smiling up at you. She is happy she was able to please you, and thankful that you made her come for the first time in her life. You curl up together in your bed, and drift off to sleep in each other's arms. You both know that you're going to have a long and happy marriage, and that your sex life is going to be great—there are so many things you want to try.

AFTERWARD, tell your partner that you had a great time leading him through this fantasy, and that you hope he had fun too! Tell him how important it is to you that he is satisfied in bed, and that you'll do whatever you can to please him.

Let him know how strong he is, and how turned on you get when he's on top of you and you can look up at his body. And remember that the smile on his face is for you, not for the mail-order bride.

Sexy Snippets

1. *She's torn between her shyness and her longing to feel your hands explore her body.*

2. *You climb on top of her, and show her how to stroke your hard penis. She's inexperienced, but her hands feel wonderful.*

3. *She was so pure, but now she's doing things she never even imagined.*

4. *She spreads her legs wide open, fucking herself shamelessly with the vibrator.*

5. *You're above her, looking down as she strokes your swollen, pulsing cock. The come blasts out of it, landing in waves on her body.*

19

THE PEEPING TOMS

Part One

OYEURISM. The word conjures up erotic thoughts of watching and being watched. It seems like we're all dying to know what goes on behind someone else's closed doors. What do our neighbors do that we don't? What do they look like when they're doing it? To see our neighbors having sex is the ultimate in forbidden witness. And there's something arousing about that intrusiveness.

In this fantasy, your partner and you are first the watchers, and then the watched. Because of the highly erotic nature of voyeurism and the very accessible plot of this fantasy, it is unlikely that you will get through both parts of it before you want to come. Therefore, we have broken the fantasy up. In Part One you are the watchers and in Part Two you are the watched.

If the weather is agreeable, choose this fantasy night to

take a walk with your partner after dark. While you are strolling along, begin to peek in the windows of the houses you walk by and wonder aloud what the inhabitants might be doing. It's always fun to peer into lit homes from the removed, darkened safety of the street, and to catch a voyeuristic snapshot glance into someone else's life.

The idea is to get yourselves in a playfully sinister mindset. If you feel comfortable, take a detour down a dark back alley or across a dark backyard on your way home. Be mischievous and ask your partner what he would think about sneaking up to someone's window—a bedroom window—and peeking inside. You don't have to actually do this, since it is the idea itself that is sexually compelling. In fact, we strongly recommend against window peeping. There'll be no time for sex if you're being fingerprinted all night.

Begin to ponder aloud what you would see if you were to play the Peeping Tom. Ask your partner what he thinks you would see. Talking about voyeurism is a terrifically smooth way to slide into this fantasy. It will give you and your partner some time alone to breathe the fresh evening air, and all the sex talk will make both of you anxious to return home to your own bedroom.

When you do get home and you're snuggled up in bed together, tell your man that you haven't been able to stop thinking about what you'd really see if you peeked into someone else's bedroom window. Tell him the idea is making you excited.

If you weren't able to go for a walk, no matter. You can start the fantasy in essentially the same way.

To set the scene, say something like:

Imagine you and I are out for an evening stroll together. It's summertime so it's still warm outside. The streets are dimly lit by streetlights and the moon is visible behind some thin clouds. We're walking down our neighborhood streets. They look so different at nighttime.

Even though you're not actually standing on the street, you can nonetheless appeal to your partner's imagination by having him visualize how different the streets are at night from how they are in the noisy hustle and bustle of day.

The houses look smaller, but the trees in the yards look bigger and the rustling of their leaves fills the night air. It's so quiet. It's strange to see our neighborhood like this—no cars, no kids, nothing. It's like another world. We're peeking in the front windows as we pass by the houses. We catch an occasional glimpse of a familiar neighbor sitting at his kitchen table or standing in her living room. We know these people well, yet they somehow seem like strangers when seen like this. It's kind of like we're intruding into their lives...

Incorporate details from your own neighborhood, and about your neighbors, to make your partner's visualization vivid.

Before we know it we've walked quite a way from our own house, further than we wanted to. We're tired, so we decided to take a shortcut through a back alley (or backyard). *We turn down the alley and we're instantly struck by how black it is. The streetlights are gone and the full moon is partly covered by clouds.*

It's so dark that we have to watch our feet as we walk, but it's kind of fun. We're laughing and trying not to trip. But we don't laugh too loudly, since we're so close to the back of the houses—we don't want to disturb anyone or draw attention to ourselves. They'd wonder what we were doing back here in the pitch black.

We realize that we've never seen any of these houses from this side before. We've only ever seen them from the street. It seems far more private back here. We almost feel like we're intruding on their personal living space. A few of the houses are designed with the master bedrooms in the lower level, and every now and then we notice a window dressing that is clearly a bedroom curtain. We start to giggle like kids when we realize we could sneak up and peek into someone's bedroom.

We dare each other to really do it. We pick a house that we can tell has a ground-level bedroom window, and we tiptoe across the dark backyard. The curtains are only half drawn, so we can see in without being seen. It's hard to be quiet since we're trying not to laugh. We can't believe we're doing this. We crouch down in apprehensive silence. Our curiosity is piqued and we're riveted to the window. We peek through it into the bedroom. There's a queen-size bed with a blue bedspread and an antique wardrobe up against a wall. There are a few toys on the floor, so we know there are kids asleep somewhere in the house. We realize suddenly that we're at the home of a couple we know, although we've never said more than "Hi" to them.

Include as many details as necessary to make the scene real to your partner. It's the small details, such as toys on the floor or the color of someone's hair, that will bring a fantasy to life in his mind. You want to do more than just bring him to orgasm—you can do that in two minutes standing against the wall if you want (and quite often, that may be exactly what you are in the mood for). But when it comes to a fantasy, you have the opportunity to spend some quality time in another world with your man, so make the most of it.

Continue with your storytelling.

Through the glass we hear the muffled sound of a door closing, and we see a man come out of what is obviously an en suite bathroom. He has a towel wrapped around his waist. He stands in the bedroom doorway for a moment, facing out into the hallway. Again we can hear muffled voices. He's talking to someone down the hall, we assume his wife. He turns around and walks toward the bed. He removes the towel and we can see him naked. He stands exposed by the bed and begins pulling back the covers. We have an unobstructed view of his cock just hanging there. It's so weird to see someone like this, in the privacy of their own bedroom, not knowing they're being watched.

You look at me quickly to gauge my reaction. You know I haven't seen another naked man since we've been together, and you're a bit uncomfortable with my seeing one now. I'm a little embarrassed but I'm also intrigued. It's more than just seeing him that's intriguing—it's the fact that he doesn't know we can see him.

The man gets into bed. He's waiting for his wife to join him, and so are we. After a few minutes she walks into the room. She's wearing a short silk nightie with spaghetti straps. It's yellow. We can't tell how long her hair is because she has it pinned up. She pushes a toy aside with her foot and jumps onto the bed. She stands up on the bed and looks down at her husband. We can hear their muffled speech and laughter. He's prompting her to do something.

Snuggle against your partner while you are telling him the prankish details of you and him crouched in the dark in someone's backyard, peeking into their bedroom window. Let him get a sense of the mischievous indecency of what you're doing, and begin to caress his body to stir his sexual interest.

Suddenly she whips the nightie over her head and we can see her standing completely naked on the bed. We pull back into the darkness reflexively, although there's no way she or her husband can see us. She's tall and seems even taller now that she's naked. Her legs are long, but her breasts are small, almost flat. Her husband grabs her ankles and makes her walk, wobbling on the bed, until she is standing directly over him. He slithers down until his face is underneath her spread legs. We can see him looking straight up at her pussy.

We're shocked but mesmerized. It's the first time we've ever seen anyone in this way. We've watched some porn movies together, but that was nothing like this. Our hearts are pounding from the forbidden excitement. I'm a little uneasy at your staring at this naked woman like this. The porn was different. It was so removed from reality that it didn't really bother me. But this is really happening, in real time, right in front of us. They're real people about to have real sex. And we're going to watch them do it.

Begin to caress your partner more urgently. Run your hands over his body lightly and teasingly. Keep pace with the increasing sexuality of the story by touching him with more pressure and insistence as the story intensifies.

I ask you if you're getting turned on by watching this, and you cautiously say, "Yes." I admit that I am, too. We watch as the woman lowers herself onto her knees right above her husband's face. He grabs her ass with both hands and pulls her down further onto his face. We have a clear view of her face as he tongues her. She has an expression of relaxed ecstasy; her eyes are closed. She's lost in it.

Touch yourself between your legs, both to arouse yourself and to let your partner know you are really getting into the fantasy.

We watch as the woman leans back on her husband until she's lying flat on her back on top of him. Her head is by his cock and she turns to lick it with her tongue. We watch, completely captivated, as he responds and begins to stiffen. He becomes fully rigid and erect within moments. He keeps licking and tonguing her pussy while she continues licking and kissing his cock. From our vantage point we can look down on their bed. It's quite a sight to see them like this. The woman's body is so exposed and open to us, her legs spread wide apart and her breasts staring up at us.

Stroke and lightly squeeze your partner's penis and testicles while you describe this part of the fantasy.

Her husband is clutching onto her thighs and eating her out. She has her head turned and is giving him a blow job. We can't believe what we're seeing and we're getting very turned on. I can feel the moisture in my panties, and even in the darkness I can see the bulge in your pants.

The man pushes his wife off of him and grabs her by her hips. He positions her on her knees, and lines himself up behind her. His cock is hard and erect. He grabs it and pushes it inside her. They start fucking doggy-style as we watch, wide-eyed and sexually enthralled. Our breathing is rapid and shallow, and our bodies are fidgeting with sexual energy.

The man holds his wife's hips as he thrusts into her. His back is arched and his head is thrown back, he's looking up at the ceiling. He's pounding her fairly hard. We can tell because every time he pushes in, we can see her body jerk forward and her small breasts shake. He's loving it. We can see his ass tighten and his hips move forward each time he pounds into her. She's loving it too. Her head is hanging down. She reaches underneath herself with one hand and begins to finger her slick clit. She lowers herself on one elbow to allow him deeper entry, and that makes him push it into her with even more force.

You are describing a potently erotic encounter, and you should keep up with your and your partner's mounting arousal by becoming more physical. Cuddle very close together, rub yourself against him, and explore his body with your hands. You can even nibble at his penis and testicles through the fabric of his clothing or underwear. Touch yourself, or take his hands and have him touch you.

We're getting extremely turned on. We look at each other with a mix of embarrassment and arousal. I can feel the hardness in your pants and I can feel my wetness soaking through my panties. A warmth is coming over my body and my nipples are hard. They're pressing against my bra, and that friction is making them burn with desire. I think how good it would feel to have your lips sucking and biting on them right now. I know you're thinking how good it would feel to have my mouth or my hands squeezing and stroking your cock until it pulses with waves of orgasm.

The woman pulls away from her husband and lies flat on her back on the bed. She pulls him toward her. He kneels between her spread legs, grabs her ankles, and lifts them up to his shoulders. She's lying there, legs open and in the air, waiting for him to penetrate her. She doesn't have to wait long. We watch as he drives his cock into her pussy again and again. He's big, but not as big as you.

We're still crouching in silence, captivated, secretly watching this couple fuck. They think they have total privacy, that not a soul in the world is aware of what they're doing or can see them doing it. We wonder if they'd feel violated and exposed if they knew they were being watched, or if they'd be turned on. We wonder how we'd feel. We're definitely turned on watching them. Our invasion into their private life is so erotic that I know very soon you're going to need to come. I can hear your breathing change; you're almost panting with excitement.

If you are not undressed yet, remove each other's clothing. Strip with abandon. Let your partner know that his release will come soon, and concentrate on massaging and caressing his penis and testicles.

The man keeps pushing his cock into his wife. He likes to watch it disappear into her pussy. We can see him looking down, watching it go in and out. The whole bed is shaking so we know he's hitting her hard. We catch glimpses as he withdraws it, and we watch as he buries it again between her long legs. We can imagine the slapping sound it must make.

I know you need to come from watching all this. I reach over and unzip your pants, then quickly begin to caress you. Your hips respond immediately and rock back and forth, pushing your cock into my hands. I tell you that we have to be very quiet and that you can't make any sound at all when you come. Your balls are firm and swollen. I can feel them beating and pulsing against my hand when I squeeze them.

There are a few ways you can steer the rest of this fantasy and your real lovemaking. In the fantasy, you can describe you and your partner as having sex outside this couple's window while watching them, and, at the same time, you can actually be having sex at home in your bed. Alternatively, in the fantasy you can describe your partner getting a blow job or a hand job, and, at the same time, you can be giving him a real one. It's entirely up to you, so do what you're in the mood for. This versatility is the reason why many of these fantasies can be revisited time and time again. They can be readily amended to suit your sexual desires of the moment.

If you choose sexual intercourse, you can say something like:

Imagine your hard-on exposed to the night air, needing to be relieved. I quickly snake out of my pants and get on my hands and knees in front of you. I present my ass to your cock and instantly feel it sink into my pussy. You bang against my body forcefully, and it seems like you're going deeper and deeper every time.

You can amend the details and dialogue to whatever sexual position you wish to adopt.

Also, be sure to revive your man's visualization.

Imagine yourself fucking me from behind. It's pitch black outside and we're in someone's backyard, peeking into their bedroom window. They're fucking each other inside and you're staring in at them, fucking me at the same time. We're actually having sex outside. We could get caught, but we can't stop ourselves. You have to come. You don't even look at me while you're fucking me. You keep your eyes glued on the couple. The woman is on her back with her legs spread in the air. The man is holding her ankles and is between her legs. He's fucking her over and over again with his cock at the same time that you're entering me with yours.

You see the man throw his head back and grind himself into his wife's pussy. He's coming. Watching him come in her makes you come too. You throw your head back like he did, and you plunge your rigid cock deep inside me, grinding against my ass. I feel your hot come spew inside me powerfully, filling my pussy. It's incredible, and I come the moment I feel it drip down over my clit.

Keep talking like this until your partner ejaculates in you, and you come.

If instead you choose to give your partner a blow job, you can say something like:

I tell you that I'm going to suck you, since I know you won't be able to walk home with your groin aching so badly. I tell you to keep your eyes glued on the couple while I suck the come out of your cock. You feel my mouth swallow your long, smooth shaft, and you feel your orgasm build as soon as my lips pass over it, sliding up and down, up and down.

Again, rejuvenate your man's visual if you choose this way to come.

Imagine you're being sucked like this. It's pitch black outside and we're in someone's backyard, peeking into their bedroom window. They're fucking each other inside and you're staring in at them, getting a blow job at the same time. I'm sucking you outside. We could get caught, but we can't stop ourselves. You have to come. You don't even look down at me while I'm doing it. You keep your eyes glued on the couple. The woman is on her back with her legs spread in the air. The man is holding her ankles and is between her legs. He's fucking her over and over again with his cock at the same time that I'm sucking you.

You see the man throw his head back and grind himself into his wife's pussy. He's coming. Watching him come in her makes you come too. You throw your head back like he did, and you plunge your rigid cock deep inside my mouth, grinding against my lips. I taste the familiar hot come quickly filling my mouth, as your hips buck. I swallow it greedily, and then come as it slides down my throat.

If you choose to give your partner a hand job, simply amend the details accordingly—and don't forget to refresh his visualization. If he is still hard after his orgasm and you have not yet come, ask him to enter you. If not, you can ask him to use his fingers or even a vibrator.

Snickering, we gather our clothes and tiptoe out of their backyard, trying to find our way in the dark. We hurry down the lamp-lit streets toward our house, not wanting to be seen or caught. We're anxious to get back to our own bed and practice what we've seen!

AFTERWARD, tell your man it was exciting to pretend you were watching a couple do it while you were doing it at the same time. Maybe there's something to be said for a little healthy, harmless voyeurism—if nobody's watching, of course. Bring him a cloth and clean him off while he relaxes and recovers. Let him know he still has Part Two to look forward to. And remember as he fades away, drunk with sexual satisfaction, that the smile on his face is for you, not for the couple you were so shamelessly spying on.

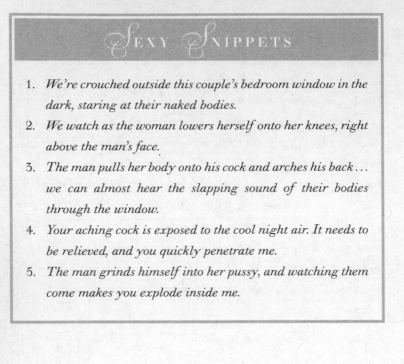

Sexy Snippets

1. *We're crouched outside this couple's bedroom window in the dark, staring at their naked bodies.*

2. *We watch as the woman lowers herself onto her knees, right above the man's face.*

3. *The man pulls her body onto his cock and arches his back... we can almost hear the slapping sound of their bodies through the window.*

4. *Your aching cock is exposed to the cool night air. It needs to be relieved, and you quickly penetrate me.*

5. *The man grinds himself into her pussy, and watching them come makes you explode inside me.*

20

THE PEEPING TOMS

Part Two

PART TWO of this fantasy picks up where Part One leaves off. That is, when you and your partner get home from your evening of serendipitous sexual spying. In this part of the fantasy, you have been very aroused by your voyeurism and have rushed home to your own bed for further sexual release. What you don't know—but will soon find out—is that the couple you were watching are in fact voyeurs themselves. And they have their sights set on the two of you.

You can begin Part Two of this fantasy by reminding your partner of Part One; review as much of it as necessary to arouse him.

After you have refreshed his memory, you can slide into Part Two by saying something like:

Imagine that by the time we get home that night we're ready to go again. We can't stop thinking of watching that couple. We can't get the images of their naked bodies out of our minds. We watched them engage in the most intensely personal and private act imaginable, and it was incredibly erotic. Our bodies are still aroused by it.

We climb into bed and start talking about it, and before we know it, I'm getting wet again and you're getting hard. We're turned on by the memory of having had sex just outside someone's bedroom window. We can't believe we really did it in their backyard like that, but they made us so hot that we had to. We could've been caught at any moment, but at the time we didn't care. The wrongness of what we did only adds to our sexual elation.

We start talking about how the woman stood over her husband so he could see her pussy, and how she lowered herself so he could eat her out. We talk about how he took her from behind and how her whole body jerked forward when he drove his cock into her. We talk about how they looked when her legs were spread in the air and he was fucking her.

They had no idea that we watched them the whole time, and that's the most arousing part. There's an intoxicating sense of erotic fascination in knowing that they were unaware of our intruding eyes, or of how turned on we were from watching them.

You and your man should begin to caress each other's body while you are telling this tale. You want to pretend that it really happened—that only minutes ago you returned home after spying on a couple having sex. You want to pretend that the pictures are still fresh in your mind and that the passion is still coursing through your bodies. Let your excitement show.

Continue with the story.

We're feeling a little devious, so I get out of bed and draw back our bedroom curtains. We've never been into exhibitionism, but right now we want to have sex with the curtains open, for the whole world to see.

Surprise your partner by getting out of bed and similarly drawing back your bedroom curtains or opening your blinds. You don't have to open them enough to actually be seen, since it's the idea itself that will turn you on. Even a slight feeling of exposure will inflame the potency of this fantasy and your shared arousal.

I get back onto the bed, but instead of lying down beside you, I stand up on the bed and remove my nightie. I stand completely naked with my legs spread above your face. I'm remembering what the woman did. I lower myself onto your face and feel your hands grab my ass cheeks. The memory of that man tonguing his wife comes to me as I feel your tongue licking my clit and darting in and out of me.

Continue to do what you are describing as happening in the fantasy. As with all fantasies, if you aren't comfortable with certain sexual acts, positions, or words, simply substitute them with ones you are more at ease with. In this fantasy, you are exploiting the sense of exhibitionism and sexual exposure more than the novelty of dirty talk or different sexual positions.

I lean back against your body, just like we watched the woman do. You grab my thighs tightly and pull me closer to your face so you can keep eating me. Your cock is by my face, and I turn my head to lick it. It springs up in an incredibly erect state. It's so swollen that it looks inches longer and much thicker than it usually does. I think about how good it will feel when you finally enter my pussy with it.

You and your partner are now pleasuring each other in a sixty-nine position.

Your perfect shaft is so sensitive that every time I wrap my mouth around it your hips push up and you moan loudly. You're thinking about that woman sucking her husband. Your eyes are closed and the images are clear and fresh in your mind... like him, you're lying flat with a woman's pussy only inches away from your face, and a hot mouth sucking on you. You're aware of our open curtains, and that knowledge makes your cock swell and throb even more.

You look at our bedroom window. Two figures are peeking in, and when they catch your eyes they retreat a little into the darkness. But you know they're still able to see, they're still watching you tongue your naked woman. They're still watching as your woman sucks your cock. We're both completely naked and available to their lustful stares.

Revive your man's visualization. It is always effective to draw back from the intensity of a specific fantasy situation, and sketch the broader picture. Hearing you say the words and describe the scene will allow your partner to get the most out of each fantasy. Not only will he be able to revel in the things you are doing to him. His arousal will be heightened by your erotic storytelling.

Imagine we're lying naked and open on our bed, sucking each other, and two strangers are watching us do it. They can see our naked bodies. They can see what we're doing to each other and how we're doing it. It's the ultimate intrusion on our privacy and our sexuality.

Under normal circumstances, you'd fly out of bed, close the curtains, and probably chase them down the street. But things are different tonight. Their presence at our bedroom window sends a wave of eroticism through your body that's almost as powerful as an actual orgasm.

I can feel the change in your body. I can feel your hips move with more urgency, and I can hear your moans become increasingly guttural. I don't know what's happening to you. You're in such an intensely aroused state that I'm not sure what to expect and I'm a little nervous. I've never seen you so worked up. I push myself off of your writhing body and face you.

You grab my face and give me a deep, passionate kiss. You whisper to me that they're watching at the window. It's that couple we were watching earlier. You don't give me a chance to pull back or reach for the sheets to cover myself. You tell me that you want them to watch. You want them to see your cock standing hard and erect, and you want them to see you fuck your naked woman. You don't give me a chance to say anything, but I'm not arguing. I see how hot you are and it makes me also want them to watch.

Spend some time giving your man a long, deeply passionate kiss. Make it the kind you enjoyed when you were dating. Explore each other through the kiss, and make it last.

You tell me to lie down on my back. You position my body so that my legs are spread open and my pussy is facing the open window. You want the couple to see the pinkness and those folds. You want them to see what you're going to fuck. You finger my clit for a while, getting me dripping wet.

Lie on your back and spread your legs, as if showing your pussy to the window. Have your partner sit on the edge of the bed in front of the window, and roll over so you can perform oral sex on him. Imagine that you are sucking on your partner in front of an envious audience, and do it like you're showing off.

Then you sit on the edge of the bed with your incredible erection pointing toward the window. You love knowing that they're staring at it, especially when it's as huge as it is right now. You love the fact that the woman is looking at it, and that she's imagining what something that big would feel like sinking into her.

You reach out and grab my head, directing it between your legs. I lean into you and bury my face in the hair of your groin, then I start sucking your dick. I like that they're watching. You put your hands on my head and push my mouth harder onto you. You want me to suck you as hard as I can while you stare at the window. No one has ever seen you getting a blow job before and you're really loving this. Every now and then you pull my mouth off of you so they get a good look at your cock.

While your man is sitting on the edge of the bed and facing the window, be sure to tell him to look at the window and imagine he can just make out the outlines of two figures peering in. He will enjoy the combined mental and physical sensations of simultaneously seeing the open window, being in the sitting position, and feeling your sucking. The result is an immediate and acute feeling of exhibitionism—a sexy twist to your lovemaking.

I know you're loving this, and I'm loving it too. I stop sucking and you push me onto my back. You kneel between my spread legs, grab my ankles, and bring them up to either side of your head. My ankles are by your ears and my pussy is open for you. We're doing the same thing we watched the couple do, so now they can watch us doing it. You remember how turned on we were, and you know they're turned on too. We've always had good sex, and I've always told you how good you are at it. Now you get to show how well you can fuck your woman.

Lie on your back and have your partner spread your legs open. Have him hold your legs high in the air while you have intercourse.

You sink your aching cock into my eagerly awaiting pussy. I look up at you, towering above me, holding my legs up and grinding your hips against me. I can't see your cock since it's buried in me. I know how good you are and I know the woman outside the window is wishing she were me right now. That makes me even hotter with desire for you.

You begin to thrust. You can feel your pubic hair against mine as your hips move back and forth, slowly at first, but then with increasing speed. Soon the room is filled with the slapping sound of your body hitting mine, hard and fast. You look down at me and see my breasts shaking from the force of your thrusts.

You look down and you can see your cock emerge from my pussy, slick with sex. You watch as it disappears just as quickly, sinking into my body again and again. Each time you bury it in me, a rush of sensation runs through and over it. We don't say a word to each other. We're both lost in the ecstasy of our fucking. The bed is rocking and so are our bodies. The slapping sound of our bodies hitting gets even louder and comes even faster as our orgasms mount.

At regular intervals, tell your partner to look at your partly open bedroom window, and to imagine there are two figures outside—they're hidden in the darkness, but they're watching every move you make. This will reestablish and exploit the intense feeling of exhibitionism. As always, let the noise you make show him how good he is making you feel.

I can feel my orgasm building. It washes over me in a hot wave of pleasure, even as you continue pounding me. Your thrusts are coming so hard and so fast now that I can't even count them or keep up with them. I know you're getting close. You're working so hard to get the come out of your cock. Suddenly you throw your head back and let out a loud moan. Your movements change from fast and desperate to slow and deliberate as the come shoots out of you in waves. It feels so good coming out that you're paralyzed until you're empty. You keep thrusting until every drop is squeezed out.

Continue talking until both of you reach orgasm.

We collapse on the bed together and look out the window. The couple is gone. They've seen what they wanted to see, and we're glad that we could return the favor. I close the curtains, and we jump out of bed to raid the fridge.

AFTERWARD, tell your man what an exceptionally good time you had during this fantasy. Tell him how incredibly good he made you feel and how you love to see him towering above you, pushing in and out of your body. Tell him nothing in the world feels as wonderful as that. Close the curtains. Bring him a snack and a glass of water. And remember that the smile on his face is for you, his fun-loving and good-spirited woman, and not for the nosy neighbors.

Sexy Snippets

1. *Imagine we're lying naked on our bed sucking each other, and strangers are watching us through our bedroom window.*
2. *You show them my pussy—you show them the soft pink folds that you're going to fuck.*
3. *You sit on the edge of the bed and lean back, letting them watch as I suck you and your cock swells and stiffens.*
4. *You know the woman outside the window is staring at your cock, wishing she were getting it.*
5. *You watch them as they stare at your hard cock plunging into my slick pussy.*

21

THE ADULT HOUSE PARTY

REMEMBER WHEN you were a teenager and a friend's parent went out of town? Inevitably, a house party followed and the teenage hormones ran free and wild. You could bet your Clearasil that the upstairs bedrooms were occupied. While heavy petting was often all that went on, an adult party filled with singles need not be as innocent. In this fantasy, your partner will find himself the lusted-after guest of an adult house party. And you get to play the hotblooded single gal who has him in her sights.

When you're in bed next to your partner, ease into this fantasy by talking about his romantic life before he met you. Flatter his ego, and talk about how the women must have been all over him.

You can ask something like:

When you were single, did you ever go to house parties? Did you ever go to one filled with a bunch of unattached women? I can imagine a house like that, especially as the night wears on. I can imagine the single women there, watching you, hoping you'll come over and talk to them. I know how women think, and they'd be thinking about you. The music is loud, the alcohol is flowing, everyone's mingling, and some are getting very close to each other. You can just tell they're aching to press their bodies against someone else. It's been a long time for some of them, including you.

At this point you should be lying beside your man, just lightly dragging your fingers across his chest. The idea is for him to close his eyes and let his mind wander, and for him to picture himself in this strange house filled with single women lusting after him.

There are so many women there, all looking for a man to touch them. They're definitely on the prowl. You have your pick. You can look around the room from one to another as each one tries to hold your gaze.

Details are important if your partner is really going to see himself in that house with those women in his mind's eye. Set the stage for this fantasy by describing what the house looks like, what the women look like, and what the other guests are doing.

Imagine you're in the living room watching everyone. People are standing very close to each other, and the women are doing their best to seduce the men. They're leaning in close, brushing against them, and laughing. You can feel yourself getting a little aroused just at the thought of what's going on around you. The alcohol is making your stomach feel warm and lowering your inhibitions.

Every once in a while you see a man and a woman go up the stairs to where the bedrooms are. The woman leads and the man follows, the bulge in his jeans obvious. You know what they're going up there for, and you begin to wonder what the chances are that you'll be as lucky.

Still lying beside your partner and whispering this into his ear, begin to work your way down to his penis just with your fingertips. You don't want to stimulate it too soon or for too long; you want this fantasy to last as long as possible. Brush across his genitals lightly, and continue down to his thighs. Make caressing circles all around them, especially his inner thighs.

Continue with the story.

You're very aware of the sensations arising in your groin in response to what's going on in the house around you, and from the thought of what you want to do with one of these girls. All your attention is focused on the steadily increasing throbbing and aching between your legs. It gets stronger every moment as you think about what is going on upstairs.

Keep touching your partner all over his body with your fingertips as you tell him this sexy story. Have him keep his eyes closed, and lead him further into the fantasy by vividly describing the developing scene for him. Take your time.

You can see two women standing across from you, by the stereo. One is a tall blonde with long hair. She's wearing dark red lipstick. The other is a brunette with short hair. They're both wearing black miniskirts with high boots. The blonde is wearing a white cotton shirt, and you can see the outline of her black bra underneath. The brunette is wearing a tank top. She's thinking about you. You can tell because her nipples are erect and showing underneath her thin shirt. You wonder if she's a little wet, too. They're giggling, and finally they come over to talk to you.

By now, your partner should be fully engrossed in this fantasy world and quite enjoying the scenery. You can keep pace with his growing sexual excitement by caressing him faster and using more pressure.

The women are standing in front of you now, chatting you up. The brunette leans over to put her drink on the table, but it's just an excuse to brush against your arm with her erect nipples. For a moment you can feel them hard against your skin. The blonde devilishly asks if you prefer blondes or brunettes. You study each girl's body shamelessly, being very bold. The drinks and your desire have made you brave.

Now it's up to your partner to decide.

The girls are being very sportive, and ask you which one of them you'd like to go upstairs with.

Take your instructions from your partner and continue the fantasy with only the girl he chooses.

Imagine that she's smiling at you, proud of herself that she won your approval, and excited about what is to come. She gazes at the bulge beginning to show between your legs, and licks her lips. She reaches out to touch it lightly, teasingly, and your cock twinges in response.

At that, touch your man directly on his penis, briefly gliding your hand along the shaft. He should still have his underwear or pajama bottoms on.

She takes your hand and leads you up the stairs. With each step you can feel your groin aching in anticipation. It almost hurts to walk. There's a long hallway at the top of the stairs with doors lining it. Some are open, and as you walk by them you can hear the sounds of people having sex inside. You can hear people moaning and beds squeaking.

Be sure to provide your partner with a good description of

the upstairs hallway and bedrooms, and of the sounds and sights therein.

You and the woman stop at one of the open doors and peek inside. There's a woman lying on her back on a bed, with her legs spread wide open. A man is kneeling above her, rubbing his cock with lubrication, and preparing to penetrate her. Both of them are naked. The man reaches down and kneads one of her breasts, then pushes his cock inside her with one fast motion. You can see her arch her back in a rush of pleasure.

The woman beside you is very turned on and you can sense her breath quickening. She continues to lead you down the hallway, looking for an empty room. Finally you find one, and she hurriedly undresses herself and you.

Now is the time to sit up and strip off your pajamas. Remove your partner's pajamas or underwear also.

She lays you roughly on the bed and crawls on top of you, kissing you hard.

Crawl on top of your partner and kiss him passionately. Really get into the role. Imagine you're a woman who's been without male contact for a long time, and now you find yourself alone with this gorgeous, naked stranger.

She tells you that she needs to feel you inside her right now, and she gets up onto her hands and knees on the bed. She tells you to fuck her fast from behind.

Get on your hands and knees quickly. Have lubrication close by to assist.

Make sure that your partner doesn't lose the image of his fantasy world as you and he begin to get more physical. Remind him where he is.

Just imagine it. You're in someone else's bedroom, on some-

one else's bed, on someone else's sheets. It's dark, and this woman you don't even know is crouched in front of you, begging you to fuck her. She's so desperate to feel your cock inside her. You can't wait to push it in and feel that aching in your groin be released. You kneel right behind her, take your cock in one hand, and drive it inside her as fast and as hard as you can.

Have your partner do just that, and heighten the thrill of penetration for both of you by moaning or grunting when you feel him enter you roughly.

It feels so good to her that she's going to come really fast. She wanted you so badly. You can see she's in ecstasy as she pushes back hard against your body and your cock, grinding her ass into your pubic hair.

Push back hard against your partner to encourage him to thrust harder into you. Remember that he is having sex with a stranger, and does not have to be as sympathetic to her feelings as he does to yours. Let him enjoy the freedom.

Continue to describe the unfolding events, refreshing his visualization.

Imagine that you look up toward the doorway and see some people watching you, just like you were watching that other couple. They just stand there, unmoving, their breathing getting quicker and quicker. You're turning them on, but the fact that they're watching you is turning you on, too. You don't mind, in fact you like it. You push as hard as you can into this girl, you don't care if it hurts her; in fact, she's liking it. You just have to get off.

It's definitely time to bring your man to orgasm, so tell him to come whenever he wants to.

Earlier in this fantasy you asked your partner to choose

which girl he wanted to go upstairs with. Be prepared for him to say both! If he does, go with it and accommodate his wishes.

If your partner wants both women, try adding a little oral sex to the fantasy. You can amend the details slightly, and say something like:

Finally you've found an empty bedroom. Both women start undressing themselves, and you. They push you roughly onto the bed. They're desperate for you and they're not going to waste any time. They throw you onto your back and spread your legs wide. Before you know it you have two women sucking on you. One is sucking your cock and the other is sucking and licking your balls. Their heads are bobbing up and down between your legs. You can't see what they're doing, but you can feel their lips and tongues moving all over your shaft and balls.

Perform oral sex with enthusiasm on your partner. Convince him that his penis is the single most delicious thing you have ever had in your mouth.

One of the girls stops and tells you that she needs to feel you inside her right now. She gets up onto her hands and knees and tells you to fuck her fast from behind.

Get on your hands and knees quickly. Make sure that your partner doesn't lose track of his fantasy as his orgasm builds. Review the scene to refresh his visualization.

Just imagine it. You're in someone else's bedroom, on someone else's bed, on someone else's sheets. It's dark, and you're with two women you don't know, both of them wanting you to fuck them. One of them is crouched in front of you, begging you to fuck her. She's so desperate to feel your cock inside her. You can't wait to push it in and feel that aching in your groin be re-

leased. You kneel right behind her, take your cock in one hand, and push it inside her as fast and as hard as you can.

While your partner is penetrating you from behind, clearly describe what the second woman is doing so that he can easily imagine the presence of another body.

The second woman is behind you. She's pushing her breasts against your back and trying to stay close to your body as you furiously fuck the first woman. You can feel her clutching your back and reaching down to squeeze your balls. You can feel her hand on your shaft as you pull out of the first girl. She's feeling your cock slide in and out.

Imagine that you look up toward the doorway, and see some people watching you, just like you were watching that other couple. Except that there's three of you. You're in a threesome, and it turns you on to realize you're being watched. You push as hard as you can into the girl, you don't care if it hurts her; in fact, she's liking it. You just have to get off. You can feel the other girl's hard nipples against your bare back. You can feel her hand exploring your cock and the other woman's pussy as you fuck each other.

Give your partner permission to come whenever he wants to. Let him know when you come by making sounds of pleasure.

Continue with the story until you are both satisfied.

Your balls contract and you come inside the woman in front of you. The second woman presses her breasts into your back and clutches your body tightly as you rock your hips into the first woman's pussy. As you come, you can feel both their bodies shudder from the strength of their own orgasms.

You fall back onto the bed in exhaustion and the women lie on either side of you, recovering. They finally get up and dress themselves, but before they leave, they scribble their phone numbers down for you. You pick your jeans up off the floor, put the numbers in a pocket, and marvel at how fun the single life can be. You head back down the stairs and rejoin the party. After all, the night's still young…

AFTERWARD, tell your man how good he made you feel and how much it turned you on to have him thrusting so hard and frantically inside you. Tell him that if you were going to pick up a man at a house party, he'd definitely be the guy you'd go after. And remember that the smile on his face is for you, not for the swinging single (or singles!) at the house party.

Sexy Snippets

1. *You follow the women up the stairs and down the hall, hearing the sounds of sex in the rooms around you.*

2. *They're desperate for you… they throw you onto your back on the bed, and spread your legs wide.*

3. *You're in someone else's bedroom, and the women are scrambling to suck your throbbing cock.*

4. *You can feel the other girl's tight nipples rub against your back as you sink into her friend's pussy.*

5. *As you come, you feel their bodies shudder from their own orgasms.*

22

SPOIL, SPA, AND SHOWER

Y HUSBAND has told me that one of his all-time favorite fantasies involves sex in the shower. It is a place where men often masturbate, and so naturally they associate it with sex. Having sex in the shower is the ultimate in pleasure for many men, so why deny it to your man? In this fantasy, your partner will have the royal treatment. He's the king of his castle, and you'll spoil him from the moment he comes in the door up to the moment he comes!

This fantasy requires a little prep time to maximize its pleasure. The idea is to spoil your man rotten before he receives his ultimate reward. Choose or arrange for an evening on which the two of you will be alone, uninterrupted. It's vital that you clear your agenda for the whole night; this fantasy is not "quickie" material. To do it right, you must set aside an entire evening that you can devote to spoiling him in every way.

Prepare your partner's favorite meal and rent his favorite movie. When he arrives, make sure all the lights are off and the house is lit only by candlelight. You want to make an impact as soon as he walks through the door, and to let him know right away that he's in for something special. Greet him wearing only a bathrobe. For a heavenly touch, invest in two new fluffy white robes—look for the big, luxurious ones that the finest spas and hotels use. If you're really ambitious, personalize them by having a unique design embroidered onto them. Put some thought into it, and choose a word or symbol that has meaning to you as a couple. It's money well spent.

Have your partner's new robe waiting for him, and ask him to put it on as soon as he gets home. He will enjoy the deluxe feel of it as much as you will, especially if his usual robe is as old and worn as some men's are. Sit your partner down on the couch; you may want to have covered it with a white sheet to make it feel a little more spa-like. Tell him to relax. Tell him you know how hard he works, and that you want to spoil him tonight. By this point, you will have already broken the routine of his usual homecoming and put a smile on his face.

Serve your man his supper on the coffee table while watching his favorite movie, or one you've both been wanting to see. Serve him his dessert, and perhaps a drink. Wait on him hand and foot. When the movie is almost over, tell him to lean back and enjoy a foot soak that you've prepared. Use Epsom salt in the water. It's inexpensive and soothing. When the movie ends, place his feet on a towel and, using a scented foot lotion—something with a peppermint or strawberry scent is particularly nice—massage each foot deeply in turn. Squeeze the heel, massage the instep, and run your fingers through the toes. There is not one person on this green earth that will not feel intoxicated by this simple but too-often overlooked pleasure. So take your time.

When you feel the moment is right, introduce some sexual energy into your man's relaxed state. Ask him to reach under the couch and see what he finds. This will be a dirty magazine or two that you have taken the liberty of providing for his pleasure. Tell him that tonight his spa attendant will attend to *all* his needs.

While it may be difficult for some women to watch as their partner becomes aroused by images of other naked women, many women enjoy pornographic images themselves, or get aroused by the effect they have on their partners. You should at least take a peek, and try it for yourself. He's in love with you, after all. As many women already know, Miss July can be an incredibly powerful sexual ally. Don't relegate your partner to catching glimpses of erotic images on the sly. Provide him with material you're okay with his seeing, and which you know will turn him on.

Continue to knead and massage your partner's feet while he looks at the pictures. Ask him to show you which ones turn him on the most, and inquire what it is about those images that he likes. Reveal the ones that turn *you* on. This discussion will foster intimacy, trust, and sexual exploration. It's also terrific foreplay.

If you wish, you can move from massaging your man's feet to caressing his genitals. In fact, you can end the fantasy here—saving the upcoming "shower sex" scene for another night—by performing oral sex on your partner and allowing him to come that way. Since many men have masturbated while looking at pornographic magazines, you can give your man the enviable experience of receiving a real blow job (or hand job) instead.

However, if you wish to proceed with the rest of the fantasy, continue as follows.

When your partner is ready to end his foot massage and put down the magazine, lead him down the darkened hallway into the candlelit bathroom. Run the shower and remove his robe. Ask him if he would like you, his personal spa attendant, to accompany him into the shower. When he says yes, step into the shower with him and begin to lather him up.

Use a loofah or sponge with a fruit-scented bath gel. This is something that most men will never, ever do for themselves, but there is no reason he will not enjoy the sensation and delicious fragrance. Many men have never used bath products such as these, so the experience may be new for him. Again, the idea is to make his shower look, feel, and smell sensually different, so that his imagination can more easily transport him into the "fantasy" shower. But even if the olfactory effect is lost on him, you'll enjoy it.

When you're lathering your man up, inject a sexy thought into your conversation. In a playful tone, say something like:

Have you ever masturbated to pictures like the ones I showed you? I've heard that lots of men masturbate in the shower. I'm sure you have, too. When you were masturbating in the shower, did you ever just wish there were someone in there with you? Did you imagine what you would do to one of those women, or what they'd do to you?

If you don't normally discuss sex so frankly, proceed slowly. Give your partner an abundance of reassuring words, touches, and glances to help him along. Immerse yourself in the pleasure of soaping your man's body up in this way, and let the water and the warmth arouse you.

Set the scene for tonight's sexual fantasy.

Imagine you're a guest at some exclusive resort and that you're getting the spa treatment. The attendant is in the shower with you, lathering you up. Picture yourself becoming more aroused as the warm soapy water slides down your body and runs between your legs. You can feel the blood pulsing to your groin, and you can feel this strange woman's hands moving all over your body. You know you're getting an erection, and you know she's going to see it. There's no way to hide it.

Continue to wash your partner all over with lots of sudsy warm water as you are saying this to him.

Finally, the woman reaches down and feels your hardness. She's obviously surprised, but she doesn't stop what she's doing. Instead, she begins to concentrate her efforts on lathering your stiffening cock and throbbing balls.

Get into a steady rhythm of pulling, pushing, and caressing your partner's penis with the rich suds. Get him as hard as you dare, and think about how good his hardness feels in your soapy hands.

You can tell that the attendant is getting turned on by touching you. She can't believe how hard you are, and she loves the way your cock feels sliding in and out of her hands, lubricated by the soapy water. She tells you that you're a very important guest, and admits that her boss told her to satisfy you in any way that you want. She's to do whatever it takes.

If you wish, you can let your partner choose how he wants to come, as follows:

She says she wants to make you come. She's staring at your cock and her hands are moving more urgently around it. It's your choice, she tells you. It's your choice how you want to come. Do you want to come on her naked body while she uses her hands? Or would you like her to kneel down in front of you and use her mouth? If you want, she can turn around and you can fuck her from behind, and come inside her. Whatever you want, she'll do. She's under orders from management to please you however you want.

Whether he chooses your hands, your mouth, or sexual intercourse, be sure to make lots of noise as he builds his momentum and comes. The sounds of sex echo in a bathroom, and that will enhance the excitement for both of you.

If you wish, *you* can direct how this fantasy ends, and how both of you will reach orgasm. For example, you can say something like:

She says she wants to make you come, but that you've turned her on so much that she has to come, too. She stands facing you, with the soapy water running over her shoulders and between her breasts. She takes your hand and places it on her pussy, gently pushing your fingers inside. She starts to rock her body as if she's fucking your fingers. Then she wraps her wet, soapy fingers around your powerful erection and starts stroking you. She uses strong, tight, slow strokes. She's trying to squeeze the come out of your cock.

Take your partner's hand and show him that you want him to use his fingers on you, while you use your hands on him. A mutual hand job is an incredibly sexy thing to do in the shower. If you've never tried it, you're in for a great time.

You continue to face each other, using your hands to mutually pleasure the other. You stare into her face, and she lets her head fall back, lost in the ecstasy of your fingers in her pussy and against her clit. She shudders, and pushes your fingers